YOUR
MIND
AT ITS
BEST

YOUR MIND AT ITS BEST

40 WAYS TO KEEP YOUR BRAIN SHARP

DAVID B. BIEBEL, DMIN,
JAMES E. DILL, MD,
AND BOBBIE DILL, RN

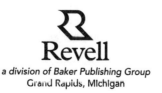

Revell

a division of Baker Publishing Group
Grand Rapids, Michigan

© 2011 by David B. Biebel, James E. Dill, and Bobbie Dill

Published by Revell
a division of Baker Publishing Group
P.O. Box 6287, Grand Rapids, MI 49516-6287
www.revellbooks.com

Printed in the United States of America

Library of Congress Cataloging-in-Publication Data
Biebel, David B.
    Your mind at its best : 40 ways to keep your brain sharp / David B. Biebel, James E. Dill, & Bobbie Dill.
        p.   cm.
    Includes bibliographical references (p.   ).
    ISBN 978-0-8007-3292-9 (pbk.)
    1. Mental health. I. Dill, James E. II. Dill, Bobbie. III. Title.
RA790.53.B44 2011
613—dc22   2010027863

Unless otherwise indicated, Scripture is taken from the Holy Bible, New International Verson®. NIV®. Copyright © 1973, 1978, 1984 by Biblica, Inc.™ Used by permission of Zondervan. All rights reserved worldwide. www.zondervan.com

Scripture marked KJV is taken from the King James Version of the Bible.

Scripture marked NASB is taken from the New American Standard Bible®, Copyright © 1960, 1962, 1963, 1968, 1971, 1972, 1973, 1975, 1977, 1995 by The Lockman Foundation. Used by permission.

Published in association with the literary agency of WordServe Literary Group, Ltd., 10152 S. Knoll Circle, Highlands Ranch, CO 80130.

11   12   13   14   15   16   17   7   6   5   4   3   2   1

green press INITIATIVE

To the memory of Dr. David B. Larson, a pioneer in the study of the relationship of faith to health, and to Dr. Harold G. Koenig, our friend, who carries forward the same banner.

Contents

Acknowledgments

We wish to thank Sue Foster, MA, LMFT, for her invaluable contribution to our effort to produce this book. We also wish to thank Gary Burlingame and Bruce Incze, whose textual contributions and research-based suggestions were so very helpful in relation to a number of chapters. In addition, we wish to thank Betsy Dill for her help in assembling the "woodpile" for the chapter "Rejoice." We could not have produced this book as well without the help of all of you. Thank you!

The Voice of This Book

When we say "we" or "our," it means that all three coauthors agree on the point in question. When one of us is describing our individual perspective or experience, we identify who is speaking in each case, by name.

Cases Cited

All the stories included in this book not identified as fictitious are true and used by permission, though most are disguised to some degree to protect the privacy of the individuals involved.

Disclaimer

Neither the authors nor the publisher are engaged in rendering medical, health, or any other kind of personal professional services in this book. Readers should consult their personal health professional before adopting any of the suggestions in this book or drawing inferences from the text. The authors and publisher specifically disclaim all responsibility for any liability, loss, or risk, personal or otherwise, which is incurred as a consequence, directly or indirectly, of the use of and/or application of any of the contents of this book.

Introduction

Most likely, your lifespan will be longer than that of your parents. But this thought comes with a caveat: As you age, you want to age gracefully, not waste away in a wheelchair somewhere, parked in front of a TV that is slowly turning the minds of everyone in that room to mush.

As our friend, neurologist William P. Cheshire Jr., MD, wrote: "The arrival of grey hairs can signify both the attainment of wisdom and the accumulation of age. In the words of Solomon of old, grey hair 'is a crown of splendor; it is attained by a righteous life' (Prov. 16:31 NIV). Grey hair is also a visible reminder of the uncertainty of maintaining mental faculties in old age. For many people, the prospect of deterioration in brain function is feared more than any other ailment of aging. Joints may give way and vision dim without eroding personal integrity. The brain, however, is essential to who we are. Its grey matter is the centerpiece of the living tapestry of personal identity."[1]

The burgeoning field of neuroscience, fueled by an amazing and increasing array of non-invasive technologies that can "see" what is going on inside your skull, is nothing short of a fourth societal revolution, according to Zach Lynch, in his compelling book, *The Neuro Revolution: How Brain Science Is Changing Our World*. The first three? Agricultural society, industrial society, and the information society. "Today we sit on the cusp of another overwhelming societal transformation, beginning to feel the liftoff of a wave potentially more dramatic than any of the three that came before. It is the emerging neurosociety," says Lynch.[2]

All of this has happened since the first whole-body magnetic resonance imaging (MRI) scan of a human being was taken on August 28, 1980, in Scotland, the first major advance in diagnostic imaging in almost 100 years (the X-ray, 1895), for which its inventors won a Nobel prize. By the early 1990s, an advancement had already occurred with MRI technology, with the development of functional magnetic resonance imaging (fMRI), which captures images not of what has happened, such as a torn cartilage, but images of activity that is going on *in real time*. Neurotechnologists can use the fMRI to detect regions of the brain that are activated when stimulated by things such as visual images. "If [neurotechnology] really works," said neuroscientist Read Montague, PhD, "then it's like nuclear energy. And these technologies are going to mature faster than people imagine. I am stunned, myself, by how well we can eavesdrop and get practical measures of what's going on in people's heads. Today, we can tell whether or not you are thinking about yourself or somebody else. . . . We wouldn't even have had this conversation ten years ago. So if it's accelerating, we're going to have a discussion of something equally surprising in just a few years."[3] Other new technologies such as the single photon emission computed tomography (SPECT) scan and the positron emission tomography (PET) scan are also used to glimpse brain health noninvasively (discounting the required injection of radioactive isotopes); computed tomography (CT) scans are sometimes used in conjunction with the latter method.

In the not too distant past, it was assumed that the older a person became, the less brain acuity he or she would possess, because the aging brain was more or less fixed or immutable. This assumption may have been based on the observation of many who developed Alzheimer's disease over time or descended gradually into dementia before expiring. Brain autopsies of those whose brains aged poorly tended to confirm the assumption, creating a self-fulfilling prognosis and a variety of myths that are in the process of being debunked. Ten of these are listed by Alvaro Fernandez in *The SharpBrains Guide to Brain Fitness*, including that: genes determine the fate of our brains; aging means automatic decline; medication is the main hope for cognitive enhancement; we will soon have a Magic Pill or General Solution to solve all our cognitive challenges; there is only one "it" in "Use it or Lose it"; all brain activities or exercises are equal, there is only one way to train your brain, we all have something called "Brain Age"; "Brain Age" can be reversed by ten, twenty, thirty years; and all human brains need the same brain training.[4]

The new technologies and brain fitness training programs are showing that the human brain is capable of lifelong learning; indeed, that neurogenesis, the generation of neurons, continues throughout life. "Learning is thought to be 'neuroprotective,'" Fernandez says. "Through neuroplasticity, learning increases connections between neurons, increases cellular metabolism, and increases the production of nerve growth factor, a substance produced by the body to help maintain and repair neurons."[5]

Complicated as some of this new information may seem, the good news is that the pillars of brain health are relatively simple and similar to the basics of good physical, emotional, relational, and spiritual health in general, with a little more focus on nutritional specifics and stress management, including meditation or prayer, physical exercise, and mental stimulation.

Think of this book as a "readers digest" compilation of information that can help you keep your mind, not lose it, as you age. We surveyed and distilled relevant and credible information from hundreds of books, articles, research findings, and internet postings in order to accomplish this.

Though a comprehensive review of the subject would take many volumes, some of them destined for obsolescence before they could reach the press, we trust you will find what we have found both helpful and hopeful as you ponder your options and opportunities for staying as sharp as possible for as long as you're privileged to share these new horizons with the rest of humanity.

—Dave, Jim, and Bobbie

| 1 |

Alter Your Brain with Prayer and Meditation

The brain needs a healthy soul and the soul needs a brain that works right.

—Daniel Amen[1]

Scientists continue to be astonished at the flood of information coming to light with new scanning technology that captures images of the living brain at work and play. Long-held beliefs about the benefits of such practices as prayer and meditation have also been proven before their very eyes. It has become an undisputed fact that prayer and meditation actually alter the brain in ways that promote physical, emotional, cognitive, and relational health. This is an exciting affirmation for those who have spent many hours talking to God and encouraging others to do the same. Meditation, also known as "mindfulness," is a practice that produces well-being and emotional balance by sculpting the brain. Dr. Daniel Amen describes meditation as a "concert state" for your brain. "By concert state I mean a relaxed body with a sharp, clear mind, much as you would experience at an exhilarating symphony. Achieving this state requires the ability to relax and focus."[2] A quick scan of the Bible produces twenty references about the practice of meditation.

In their 2009 book, *How God Changes Your Brain*, Dr. Andrew Newberg and Mark Robert Waldman illustrate how spiritual practices like intense prayer and/or meditation improve memory, cognition, and compassion while suppressing undesirable responses like anger, depression, and anxiety. They explain how these practices work directly on the brain circuits. For instance, the anterior cingulate in the brain is identified as our "neurological heart" and provides communication between the frontal lobe (thoughts and behavior) and the limbic system (feelings and emotions). The more active our anterior cingulate, the more empathy we will have and the less likely we will be to react with fear and anger. Prayer and meditation help us to become more compassionate![3]

Gus was a participant in one of Newberg and Waldman's studies on the benefits of meditation. He had come to the clinic because of concerns about his faltering brain, but had never meditated a day in his life. He overcame his skepticism and was determined to give it a try. He was prescribed a routine of twelve minutes of mindfulness exercises a day. "After only eight weeks of practice his brain was scanned and showed remarkable increase of neural activity in the prefrontal cortex, an area involved in helping to maintain a clear, focused attention upon a task. In addition, the anterior cingulate was also activated which is involved with emotional regulation, learning, and memory and is particularly vulnerable to the aging process. The anterior cingulate plays a major role in lowering anxiety and irritability and also enhances social awareness."[4]

Intense prayer has similar effects upon our brain. Five minutes once a week will have little effect, but people who make prayer a meaningful part of their day actually train and modify their brain in a way that is believed to be permanent. The more one believes in what he or she is praying about, the stronger the response will be. Catholic nuns who had practiced "centering prayer" for a minimum of fifteen years were studied. The goal of centering prayer is to get in touch with the heart of God, which brings about a sense of peace, comfort, and compassion. The brain scans found that intense prayer brought about significant neurological changes that were very different from how the brain usually works.[5]

Numerous studies have verified that even as young children we begin to form a mental image of who God is. This might begin, for example, on our very first Christmas when we are surrounded with all kinds of visual, auditory, and olfactory stimuli, which we connect with Jesus' birthday. Since as young children we think in pictures and cannot as yet form abstract thoughts, our view of God and Jesus is formed by what we experience and what we hear the adults around us saying. The whole experience of reading the Christmas story, setting up the manger, making the special cookies, the arrival of grandparents laden with gifts, the beautiful tree, and the singing of carols all hopefully form positive images of a loving Father God.

This early view then continues to evolve as we grow and have additional positive experiences related to the character of God. Studies have shown that if a person was exposed to God or Jesus as a young child, a memory circuit is established and is triggered each time the person has similar experiences or even just thinks about God. Therefore, prayer or meditations that center on a loving God strengthen that early neuronal pathway and pave the way toward a more "adult" experience of security and serenity that are the best protection from the brain-threatening anxieties and stresses that often accompany life's inevitable difficulties. We just love that Old Testament promise: "Thou wilt keep him in perfect peace, whose mind is stayed on thee: because he trusteth in thee" (Isa. 26:3 KJV).

| 2 |

Ask: Is It Alzheimer's, Aging, or Stress?

Our brain creates our life: perception, movement, thought and emotion, memories, speech and intelligence are features of this extraordinary and most complex organ.

—Author unknown[1]

We treasure our brain and all its "performances"; that is why when we begin to detect some slips and slides in memory we panic and maybe even wonder if we could have Alzheimer's. To avoid unnecessary worry and to guard our brain health it is important to know the facts and when, or if, we need to get a brain check-up. The great majority of the time when we notice memory problems it is due to the way we process information, increased stress, or even the natural process of aging.

Memory lapses are often caused by a lack of stimulation or being fully engaged in life, which can result in a lag in forming new brain cells and pathways. Forgetting something we just learned yesterday is frustrating, but it's even worse when we can't remember something we've known for years! What we're trying to recall seems to be "on the tip of our tongue," but the brain's search for the right file in the neuronal archives turns up empty. Of course the harder we try to make ourselves remember, the more stubborn our "search engine" becomes. This plight not only disturbs us, but it can affect our friends as we turn to them with a plea for help only to find that they, too, have developed "amnesia" in relation to what our Googling brain is searching for. When this occurs, our stress level may increase: for example, if we're late for an important appointment, and we need to call the other person, but we simply can't remember that telephone number. Avis can't help us here, either, since the harder we try, the worse it gets.

The phenomenon behind these occurrences takes place in the frontal lobe of our brain, which is very sensitive to stress hormones. When the frontal lobe (the keeper of stored memories) senses fight or flight situations, it shuts down to allow lower brain functions to use the energy. In other words, if our brain detects a dangerous or stressful situation it automatically ramps up the areas needed to keep us safe, in which case remembering our aunt's address is no longer a priority. Of course that needed piece of information often pops back into our mind when it is no longer needed and we are working in the garden or drifting off to sleep! Dave had this experience recently, when he and his sister were visiting during a family reunion, and she was trying to recall the name of the fire chief in their town when they were kids. Neither could remember, hard as they tried to do so. But when Dave was drifting off to sleep that very night, Mr. Buchanan's name came to his mind like magic.

Perhaps you can relate to the following excerpts from a *New York Times* description of one couple's apprehensions about staying sharp mentally:

> It was 12:30 and Natalie and Mel Gordon were having their lunch at a bustling diner on the Upper East Side. They live in Flushing, Queens; married 55 years, and are full of vigor. Mrs. Gordon is 75 and used to be a social worker in a nursing home. Mr. Gordon is 80. Before retiring, he worked in advertising and then taught high school English.
>
> "We joke about having a 'senior moment,' the buzz phrase for forgetting something, but it's also serious," Mrs. Gordon said meditatively. "Because we all fear Alzheimer's or something that will affect us mentally.
>
> "The big concern for me is, will I recognize it when it begins," Mrs. Gordon said. "If I tell a joke a second time to the same people, is that it? The fear for me is, will I not recognize it and then slip into a condition where I will not be able to deal with my family and those I love."
>
> The Gordons are active people. They volunteer. They go out a good deal. They support each other. They make lists galore. She has a special place where she stashes an extra comb for when he loses his. They belong to a book discussion group, and after the views on the book are offered, the members typically drift into what they teasingly call their "organ recitals," when they rattle off capsule updates on their ailments. . . . The other day during one of the organ recitals, the Gordons went ahead and broached the topic. Everyone chimed in. They all expressed their fears.[2]

As humorous as memory laments can be, situations turn serious when memory lapses worsen or are combined with other symptoms. Dementia, including Alzheimer's, results in a gradual loss of intellectual function. Symptoms include memory loss, problems with focus, language, and problem solving skills, difficulty controlling emotions and moods, and personality changes. Alzheimer's, the thief of memory, usually targets the hippocampus first and then spreads to other areas of the brain, slowly killing brain cells and rendering its victim incapacitated. Amyloid, a protein that is produced in the small intestine, is secreted into the bloodstream. When this toxic substance is deposited in the brain it can cause inflammation and nerve cell tangles. In 2009, a multi-center research team made a critically important discovery. Dr. William Klein and colleagues proved that "Oleocanthal, a compound found in extra-virgin olive oil, alters the structure of neurotoxic proteins believed to contribute to the debilitating effects of Alzheimer's disease. This structural change impedes the proteins' ability to damage brain nerve cells."[3] Oleocanthal, a different protein than Amyloid, binds to nerve cell synapses and blocks Amyloid binding, which is thought to be the crucial first step that triggers Alzheimer's. If this finding holds true when tested in upcoming clinical trials it could lead to successful prevention and treatment for this debilitating and incurable disease!

Realizing there is hope will make it easier for people like the Gordons to muster up the courage to take the specific tests at the doctor's office to determine if symptoms are Alzheimer's, aging, or stress. In the past it was believed that genes were the key instigator, but now there are many more theories about what contributes to the development of Alzheimer's. Among them are such things as immune dysfunction, metabolic conditions including obesity, overwhelming stress such as PTSD, and environmental toxins. Recently, saturated fat specifically was implicated when it was discovered that saturated fat can damage the blood vessel lining in the brain, thereby allowing buildup of the protein Amyloid.[4]

Scientists have shown that in actuality only about 4 percent of the population between ages sixty to seventy-four develop Alzheimer's. But the figure jumps to almost 50 percent after age 85.[5] Dr. William R. Markesbery and his colleagues examined numerous patients at the time of their death and were astonished to find that about half of a large group of elderly well-educated people with no signs of intellectual decline at their deaths actually had numerous plaques and tangles warranting a diagnosis of Alzheimer's!

How could this happen? Most experts believe that those with damaged brains but few or no symptoms were able to "recruit" healthy neurons and brain circuits in order to function normally.[6] In addition, it has been noticed that seniors who exercise and eat a Mediterranean-style diet seem to be at lower risk for Alzheimer's. This was recently proven by researchers at Columbia University when 1,880 septuagenarian New Yorkers were studied, and those who followed the healthiest diets were 40 percent less likely to develop Alzheimer's. In addition, those who got the most exercise were 37 percent less likely to develop the disease. The greatest benefit occurred for those who both ate healthfully and remained active. Those who scored high in *both areas* were 59 percent less likely to develop Alzheimer's![7]

If you are concerned about developing Alzheimer's, this one finding simply cannot be ignored. On the other hand, if you want to develop some or all of the following symptoms, then change nothing and leave your brain's future to chance:

1. Memory changes that disrupt daily life.
2. Challenges in planning or solving problems.
3. Difficulty completing familiar tasks.
4. Confusion with time or place.

5. Trouble understanding visual images and spatial relationships.
6. New problems with speaking or writing.
7. Misplacing things and losing the ability to retrace steps.
8. Decreased or poor judgment.
9. Withdrawal from work or social activities.
10. Changes in mood and personality.[8]

| 3 |

Avoid Dirty Water

Once we can secure access to clean water and adequate sanitation facilities for all people, irrespective of the difference in their living conditions, a huge battle against all kinds of diseases will be won.

—Dr. Lee Jong-wook, Director-General, World Health Organization[1]

Okay. You're standing on that scale again, convinced it must be off by at least ten pounds of ugly fat. But did you know that 60–70 percent of your total weight is water? About 90 percent of your blood is water. About 75 percent of your brain is water. Water is essential for your life. But too much water (water intoxication) as well as too little water (dehydration) can affect your brain and in severe cases even lead to death. That is why it is crucial to drink sufficient amounts of clean water every day and to avoid contaminated water as much as possible.

Children, especially, need clean water, since they are often more vulnerable than adults to problems with drinking water because their bodies and brains are developing. This need has led to testing tap water in schools and daycare centers.[2] Problems with unclean water have occurred across the country for a variety of reasons: corroded plumbing of large school buildings, poor water quality of country schools that obtain water from private wells, and under-maintained conditions of large and small daycare centers. These conditions can result in elevated levels of lead and copper. Concerned parents should first inquire with the educational facility's persons in charge. Some water testing may have already been done. Certified laboratories can be contacted to provide water testing, if needed. In all cases, there should be recent information about the safety of the tap water. Additional concerns can always be directed to the state's environmental health officers or the EPA (EPA Safe Drinking Water Hotline 1-800-426-4791).

Do you take your tap water for granted? That is, do you expect that every time you turn on the kitchen faucet, clean, drinkable water will come flowing out? Do you also take water for granted when you bathe and shower—when you immerse yourself beneath the safe, warm water and wash your face? This is true for most Americans, even though a 2009 report found that bathroom shower heads are often a breeding ground for bacteria.[3]

Worldwide, many people would be happy just to have a shower head to sanitize; instead, they don't even have access to safe, clean water, if they have running water at all. In 2004, the World Health Organization reported that over one million people die every year from water-related diseases, most of them being children under five years of age in countries where safe water and sanitation are lacking. So if you're traveling abroad, you need to check with travel experts about the safety of the tap water at your destination, and if necessary, take along appropriate treatment options or filtration systems to protect your health in general, and your brain in particular.[4]

We (Bobbie and Jim) can attest to this when, on a recent medical trip to American Samoa after the tsunami, contaminated water was a significant problem. Not only was it critical to remember never to drink from the faucet or use tap water while brushing teeth, but we had to come up with creative solutions while seeing patients in clinic and when cooking meals. It was hard to convince the Samoan children who love to swim that their favorite swimming beach was now off limits. It was always a priority to remind ourselves and the Pacific Islanders to stay hydrated, counteracting the effects of the hot, tropical climate. We returned home with a renewed sense of thanksgiving for our abundant supply of clean water.

Even water that has been treated and comes out of your tap can have contaminants that affect your health. Although your water supplier may be doing everything it can to provide you with safe tap water, chemicals can enter your water in your own home. Lead is one such contaminant[5] and is of particular concern for pregnant women and young children. Lead poisoning can damage the nervous system and brain. Although lead exposure is more common from paint and dust, lead can come from leaded pipe and solder in your home water system.

Animals and birds, as well as humans, contaminate water. You can get sick from drinking water from a creek even though the creek is way up in the mountains, far away from any human activity. Drinking contaminated water can introduce parasites to your body. Most of these cause gastronomical illness until treated, but some can affect the brain.[6]

You don't have to *drink* bad water to get sick. Recreational water illnesses, according to the U.S. Centers for Disease Control and Prevention, are illnesses that are spread by swallowing, breathing, or having contact with contaminated water from swimming pools, spas, lakes, rivers, or oceans.[7] These infections can cause neurologic problems. Children, pregnant women, and people with compromised immune systems are more at risk if they acquire such an infection.

This true story illustrates some of the potential confusion related to clean water:

> A concerned mother called her water company. "Is it safe for my son to drink our tap water?" she asked.
>
> "May I ask why you are asking that question?" the water scientist replied.
>
> "My son's doctor told us that he should avoid the tap water."
>
> "Was there a reason your doctor told you to avoid the tap water?"
>
> "My son is still on drugs that make him immunosuppressed. He had a heart operation. The heart doctor gave us a long list of things to do and not to do. My son wants to stay active and him being a teenager, there are only so many dos and don'ts I will be able to hold him to."
>
> "Did the doctor put the need to avoid tap water high on his list?"
>
> "Yes, she did."
>
> "I'm curious as to what activities your son wants to stay involved with."
>
> "Well, he likes to swim in the local public swimming pool."
>
> "Did the doctor tell you to avoid swimming in public swimming pools?"
>
> "No, she did not."

"I understand your concern for your son and your challenge in holding him to a list of dos and don'ts," the scientist replied. "But I would suggest that you give your doctor a call. With what I know about the health risks of public swimming pools, you might want to ask the doctor if that should be more important than avoiding the tap water, which actually poses no risk at all."

The mom did call the heart doctor and she did rearrange the priorities of what her son should avoid to reduce his risks. But the doctor was embarrassed. She called the water company and told them they should not be giving advice to her patients. The bottom line is that while doctors may be experts in the human body, they do not always understand the risks associated with drinking water and recreation in water.

Water is essential for the enjoyment of life, and clean water is essential for a healthy life. You need to maintain a healthy lifestyle that includes regular consumption of safe water. Since you also use water to shower and bathe, to wash your hands, and to wash your food and kitchenware, you need to make sure that your water is clean and safe.

How do you know if your water is safe? The U.S. Environmental Protection Agency oversees the nation's standards for the quality of tap water when that water comes from a water supply other than a private well or spring. The regulations are enforced by most state environmental agencies. Since 1974, over eighty different contaminants have been regulated. Public water suppliers are required to provide an annual water quality report called a Consumer Confidence Report. This report tells you what contaminants are found in the water you drink, and whether they are found at levels that you should be concerned about. If you are still concerned about the quality of your tap water, you can find a certified laboratory to test your water for the contaminants of concern in your area by contacting your state's environmental health department. And before you run to the store to load up on bottled water, check with the EPA's Water Health Series at www.epa.gov/safewater or call the Safer Drinking Water hotline at 1-800-426-4791 to obtain more information on bottled water, which may contain similar levels of the same contaminants found in tap water around the country.

| 4 |

Become a Lifelong Learner

The brain wants to learn. It wants to be engaged as a learning machine.

—Dr. Michael Merzenich[1]

You may have learned in school that the number of brain cells one has is fixed. With this in mind, educators encouraged us to act with care to preserve whatever number of brain cells we had. At the same time, this teaching may have created a sense of futility that our brainpower was fixed and that, as we aged, the best we could do would be to limit our losses. For example, how many times have you heard that a single alcoholic drink kills X number of brain cells, the implication being that if you weren't really careful you might pickle your brain by the time you were fifty (assuming you did take that occasional drink *and* that the brain could not produce new cells).

Today we know that the brain is very capable of growth even into our senior years.[2] And there is even more good news. Cognitive performance in older adults appears to be improving over time. A recent study with a United States and United Kingdom sample found that older people today show less cognitive impairment than earlier cohorts. Because of improvements in medicine, health care, and other social factors, many people do perform well in old age and continue to learn new skills.[3] One key to retaining brain health into our later years seems to be to keep learning. Learning stimulates the brain. To date, no particular regime of learning is shown to be better than another, so feel free to pursue that lifelong passion. Commit your brain to learning what is fun and satisfying.

Our friend Bruce Incze reports, "My father immigrated to this country in 1951. He was a poor war refugee, who brought with him his twelve-pound, 1937 Remington Junior typewriter, equipped with Hungarian as well as English characters. Dad was and is a writer. His typewriter is now an heirloom and is still in functional order. Being a passionate writer and a practical man, at sixty-five years of age, he realized that learning to word process on a computer would benefit his writing endeavors. Thus, his passion (writing) and a need for learning (word processing) were combined. Learning to operate a computer was slow and frustrating at first, but the brain did not object to the workout. At sixty-nine years of age, he was awarded the Gold Medal for *Footprints of Destiny Lane*[4] by the Árpád Academy of Arts and Sciences, a society for the preservation of Hungarian culture. Since then, Dad has learned one operating system after another. He even had to abandon his favorite word processing software as it became obsolete. This was somewhat traumatic as no other word processing program supports the ease of bilingual writing he had come to master. Given this new obstacle, why persevere? Because he still had a fire in the belly to write. He has published many non-commercial books since then. Even today, he continues to learn new computer technologies, at ninety-four years of age. (He is intentional to say, 'I am ninety-four years of age' and not 'I am ninety-four years old.') He has moments of frustration, but he learns new skills because they are needed to express his passion through writing. To this day, he remains as sharp as a tack and a delight to engage in conversation."

And then there is Bobbie's Aunt Nancy, now in her eighties and still young at heart. Nancy had been an avid sailor in her youth and spent many happy hours out on the water with her husband, Pete, a former Navy man. Her spirit of adventure kept her intent upon living an active lifestyle. A sailing adventure package for seniors caught her attention and she soon had connected with others of like mind and was ready to set sail. She loves to relate her adventures as she and her seven new friends sailed a forty-eight-foot-long Catamaran around the islands off the Bahamas, under the guidance of a fun-loving crew of three. As you can imagine, many of the old brain connections made early in life were re-activated and strengthened amid laughter and the thrill of adventure.

Without doubt, your brain is a resilient organ. Even if you have allowed your brain to become something of a couch potato, it is never too late to try something new. In the largest controlled clinical trial to date, memory, concentration, and problem-solving skills of healthy adults ages sixty-five and older were improved by cognitive training.[5]

The brain is capable of improved health. Just like someone can make a commitment to losing weight and improving fitness, one can commit to preserving and improving brainpower. And like physical exercise, no one else can do it for you. Since learning is a means of promoting brain health, find a hobby that works the brain. Exploring a new hobby will often put you in contact with new acquaintances, creating new social circles.

Dave's friend Len has been "retired" for some time, but he has kept his brain sharp by immersing himself continually in new hobby-type engagements, from building a huge model train layout to scale, building ships to scale in a bottle, tackling extremely detailed woodworking, and learning digital photography and photo editing. Len never seems to tire of trying new things.

Remember, your brain wants to learn. Find an activity where learning is play and then let your brain romp around in that field.

| 5 |

Brain Safe Your Home

Minds, like bodies, will often fall into a pimpled, ill-conditioned state from mere excess of comfort.

—Charles Dickens

Your home may be cozy, full of toys and good books. You might have DVD movies with a wide-screen TV. You might have a hot tub in which to unwind after a hard day at work, or a big kitchen in which to relax by preparing and cooking gourmet dinners. But your home may also be filled with safety and health hazards! Have you ever inspected your home using a safety checklist to see how many hazards you might find?

You may spend half of your life at work or school, but the other half you spend at home. Workplaces have safety rules with inspections and warnings for workers. How many homes have you been in where safety rules were posted? Many injuries and illnesses occur in the home environment. These include head injuries from accidental falls, lead poisoning of children, and poisoning from inhaling or ingesting a variety of common substances—all of which can be prevented with common sense and good housekeeping. Use your good mind to protect your brain from injury!

Chemicals may be found throughout your home—bleach, ammonia, roach traps, nail polish remover, isopropyl alcohol, drain cleaner, carpet cleaner, paints, paint thinners, gasoline, glues, and other adhesives. Serious consequences can result from exposure to pesticides and their residues, indoor toxicants, tobacco smoke, solvents, and combustion gases such as carbon monoxide. Read the labels of all the chemicals you store in and around your house. You may be surprised by what you find. Labels contain important information such as warnings to keep them out of reach of children. This does not mean you should get rid of all these chemicals. Rather, you should respect them for what they can do if they are not handled and stored properly.

Carbon monoxide is a very dangerous gas, partly because it is colorless and odorless—it is a silent killer.[1] Whenever a gas oven or heater or automobile is running in an enclosed space there can be danger from carbon monoxide poisoning. Early symptoms can include headache and dizziness. Carbon monoxide poisoning affects the heart, lungs, and brain. It interferes with the heart and brain's ability to get oxygen. Babies, infants, and the elderly are most vulnerable. But there is a way to protect yourself. You can install carbon monoxide detectors, similar to smoke detectors, in your home.

According to the U.S. Centers for Disease Control and Prevention, approximately 250,000 children aged one to five years have blood lead levels greater than the level at which action should be taken.[2] Lead poisoning can occur with no obvious symptoms or warning signs. However, children's blood lead levels can be checked. Lead poisoning is preventable. Lead-based paint and lead-contaminated dust are major sources of exposure even though lead-based paint was banned in 1978 in the United States. Old homes deteriorate and the lead paint peels off and becomes dust around the house where children play. Children under the age of six years old are at greatest risk because of the effect of lead on their development. Other sources of lead exist, such as contaminated soil and toys, jewelry, cookware, and cosmetics that contain lead.

Other things in your home can also pose a risk to children or adolescents, including access to electrical outlets (for young children), glues and other adhesives used in hobbies, alcohol that is made for consumption, prescription drugs that affect the brain, and even—hard to believe—your office supplies, including various adhesives, solvents, even "canned air."

Humorous as it may sound, Dave was discussing this chapter with his father, who grew up in the late 1930s and '40s, and his dad mentioned that there was no warning on the glue that he and his friends used to make models in those days, so they sniffed it and they ate it—thankfully with no long-term complications. But another example from Dave's life isn't quite so humorous. Some time ago, a distant relative who was around twenty years old tried to dull the pain that plagued him by sniffing glue and gasoline. At a point when he was obviously not in his right mind, he took his Model 94 30-30 carbine rifle down to the general store in the town where he lived, with the ultimate result being his confrontation with an array of state troopers, all of whom had their crosshairs fixed on his chest. With all the warnings, he knew that if he lifted his own rifle even a little, to challenge his adversaries, they would shoot. He did; and they did. And the result was an epitaph that might have been very different.

You may think that such a thing could never happen to you or your family, but go into your bathroom closet and count the prescription drugs (and other drugs) that a person could use to commit suicide if he wanted to do so. Yes, even Christian kids can reach that sense of hopelessness when their brain is not functioning properly and reality is out of reach for the moment.[3] Your teenage son or daughter lives in a highly charged environment, where images of death permeate their music, and examples of early death of their icons suggest that this is a good way to go. You should assume that your teenage kids already know what drugs are in your medicine chest, and how much of each type or a combination of them would achieve the desired effect. Without doubt, for one reason or another, some kids want to get "high."

Let's just think of Kyle for example, in the words of his own brokenhearted policeman father:

> On March first I left for work at 10 p.m. At 11 p.m. my wife went down and kissed Kyle goodnight. At 5:30 a.m. the next morning Kathy went downstairs to wake Kyle up for school, before she left for work. He was sitting up in bed with his legs crossed and his head leaning over. She called to him a few times to get up. He didn't move. He would sometimes tease her like this and pretend he fell back asleep. He was never easy to get up. She went in and shook his arm. He fell over. He was pale white and had the straw from the Dust Off can coming out of his mouth. He had the new can of Dust Off in his hands. Kyle was dead.
>
> I am a police officer and I had never heard of this. My wife is a nurse and she had never heard of this. We later found out from the coroner, after the autopsy, that only the propellant from the can of Dust Off was in his system. No other drugs. Kyle had died between midnight and 1 a.m.
>
> I found out that using Dust Off is being done mostly by kids ages nine through fifteen. They even have a name for

it. It's called dusting. A takeoff from the Dust Off name. It gives them a slight high for about ten seconds. It makes them dizzy. A boy who lives down the street from us showed Kyle how to do this about a month before. Kyle showed his best friend. Told him it was cool and it couldn't hurt you. It's just compressed air. It can't hurt you. . . .

Kyle was wrong.[4]

The fact is, there are probably a dozen or more things in your home right now that could seriously injure or even kill you or your kids. But you can protect yourself and your family. Here are some things to do in your house to help protect and maintain a healthy brain:

- Check for things that could lead to accidents, such as uneven thresholds between rooms, carpet that is not fixed in place, slippery tiles, steps without railings to hold on to, cords that run across the floor, and places where loose items may spill out onto the floor.
- Check for chemicals such as cleaning supplies that might be stored under the sink or in a closet, paints and varnishes and related chemicals, insecticides, and bleach near the washing machine. Store these in safe places, such as cabinets that can be locked. Make sure you take notice of the warnings on the labels.
- When you paint or use solvents, always provide good ventilation.
- Make sure that heaters, ovens, and stoves are working properly. Improperly operating combustion devices can fill the home with dangerous gases.
- Place smoke alarms and carbon monoxide detectors throughout the house.
- Check all items that a child comes in contact with for possible lead content. Make sure old paint and dust are

cleaned away. Clean children's hands when they come in from playing outside.

- Make sure you do not have old lead pipes in your house or in the service line that brings water to your house from the street main if you are supplied by a public water system.
- Restrict access to all prescription medications.
- If small children sometimes visit, be sure your outlets are covered.
- Keep all your office supplies in a safe place.
- Remain sensitive and alert to allergies that might be developing in your family.
- Stay alert to communications between your teenage kids and their friends, in relation to various methods to "get high." Better to offend them than to bury them.

Make safety and health checks of your home environment. Too many accidents happen every year in the home. You shouldn't have to wear a hardhat, safety shoes, or a mask at home! Your home should be a safe and healthy place for you and your family, where you can also show hospitality to friends and strangers.

| 6 |

Discover Something

If you could use a video camera to watch the brain respond to experiences, I have no doubt you would see it growing, retracting, reshaping.

—Larry Squire M.D., Professor of Neuroscience, University of California at San Diego[1]

Fantastic images of the brain revealed by positron-emission tomography (PET) and MRI scans amaze and delight researchers as they study the brain. Not only can they closely inspect the brain's anatomy, but they can watch as different areas light up in brilliant colors as people are engaged in various activities. This knowledge has been filtering out to interested learners everywhere as we grasp the amazing truth that our brain is growing and changing moment by moment. The old idea that our brain is only a stagnant machine hidden away in our skull and slowly wearing out has given way to the startling truth that our brain, among other feats,

41

grows new neuronal pathways in response to mental challenges. The process of discovery is one of these invigorating challenges. And it brings an added benefit, too—the joy of finding something new.

Deep in our gray matter is an area with a catchy name, anterior cingulate cortex, that has been recently dubbed the "eureka circuits." It is here that hundreds of brain cells called neurons become active when we are in the process of exploring. Scientists at the University of Lyon in France did an experiment that involved monkeys, who were presented with a choice of touch keys on a computer screen and encouraged to spend time exploring which ones resulted in producing a desired juice drink. Then they were given a few seconds to take full advantage of their discovery and get more drinks. As they did, hundreds of neurons lit up as researchers monitored their brain activity. The importance of this discovery helped the scientists understand the change that takes place as we find the sought-after item, stop our exploring behavior, and actually begin taking advantage of the find.[2]

We have all had our "aha" moments, which usually materialize without warning when we change how we perceive a situation. Sometimes it brings a solution to a gnarly problem; or it could be suddenly recognizing a face or even finally getting a joke! As simple as these discoveries may seem, they actually are born out of the culmination of intense and complex changes in the brain that require a lot more neural resources than ordinary analytical thinking. Dr. Mark Wheeler, a psychologist at the University of Pittsburgh, was the first to map the decision-making and evidence-gathering process prior to the actual "eureka" moment, using high tech brain-scanning equipment. He found that our brain is actually highly engaged when our mind is *wandering* and is working quite hard right before this moment of insight.[3]

Researchers report that a happy, serene "mental life" is fertile ground for eureka moments. Newton's moment of discovery about gravity occurred in an orchard as he watched an apple fall from a tree. Descartes was in bed watching flies on his ceiling when the ideas foundational to "Cartesian coordinates" came to him. His development of these ideas revolutionized mathematics by providing a systematic link between Euclidean geometry and algebra. Archimedes was about to take a bath. When he stepped in, he noticed that the water level rose, and suddenly he realized that the volume of water displaced must equal the volume of the part of his body that was submerged. The implication was that the volume of irregular objects (such as one's leg) could be calculated with precision, a problem that previously had seemed unsolvable. The legend says that Archimedes was so excited by his discovery that he leapt from the tub and then "streaked" through the streets of Syracuse, naked, shouting "Eureka! I've got it."

All around us, we can see others experiencing the excitement and joy of discovery. Think of a child's Easter egg hunt. The child doesn't even have to be an "egg lover" to become totally involved in the challenge of the hunt. Each child is on high alert as they scramble and climb and dive for those hidden colored eggs! Treasure hunts have the same allure, even for adults, some of whom end up turning their avocation into a vocation.

For example, just around the corner from Dave's home in Florida is Mel Fisher's Treasures—Museum and Gift Shop. One might think such a place to be just another tourist trap, but here's a little of the story of someone who used every day to discover something new, as posted on the website http://www.melfisher.com:

> Mel Fisher, a dreamer, a visionary, a legend and most importantly, the World's Greatest Treasure Hunter! Mel Fisher

43

did what many have not—he realized his dream during his lifetime. Every day he insisted, "Today's the Day!" His mantra continues to inspire the search for the rest of the treasure from the *Nuestra Senora de Atocha* and the *Santa Margarita*, the Spanish galleons that sank during a hurricane on September 6, 1622, near Key West, Florida.

The $450 million dollar treasure cache or "*Atocha* Mother Lode" would be found on that momentous day, July 20, 1985. Over 40 tons of silver and gold were located including over 100,000 Spanish silver coins known as "Pieces of Eight," gold coins, Columbian emeralds, silver and gold artifacts and over 1000 silver bars.[4]

There are many discovery museums scattered about our country where children as well as adults can spend hours experiencing "eureka moments." Want to know how a wave is made? Or how about a tornado? Have you always wondered how the heart squeezes blood to all parts of your body? You can almost feel the brain-jogging benefits as you go from exhibit to exhibit.

I (Jim) have always been fascinated by technology and am challenged by the new gadgets that are added to our repertoire to help people. Several years ago I was searching for the cause of a patient's abdominal pain, which had escaped detection by the usual tests. I was convinced that there was something amiss and had prayed for guidance. This day I was using a fairly new ultrasound invention that allowed me to not only see the walls of the stomach but also *through* the stomach wall. As I searched for the abnormality, I suddenly began to see small reflecting particles light up in the area of the gall bladder. Upon further scrutiny it was apparent that these were actually tiny pieces of sludge on their way to becoming stones not yet large enough to show up on our usual tests. But it was enough to cause the chronic abdominal pain the

patient had been experiencing. It was a moment of thankful-
ness to the Great Physician as well as satisfaction that I was
able to assure this patient that there was a cause and a cure
for her chronic pain. The pain was certainly not "all in her
head" as she had begun to fear. That experience led to many
more days of discovery as I searched for a hidden cause for
the problems my patients were experiencing.

Discovery's benefits are not limited to what they do for
you; you can also gain benefits by joining in the excitement
of others as they make their discoveries. One of the many
joys of being a grandparent is getting that phone call from
your grandchild relating their own latest discovery. Our then
five-year-old granddaughter had just moved to Florida when
on one of her first trips to the beach she called, her voice
full of excitement. "Nana, guess what I found? The ocean is
full of baby seahorses!" she exclaimed, too thrilled to take
a breath. "They are swimming all around and look just like
real horses except they have a mermaid tail . . . and they
don't even bite!" This day of discovery ushered in a great
learning experience for all of us as we learned more about
Florida marine life.

As Ralph Waldo Emerson assured us, "We are all inventors,
sailing out on a voyage of discovery; guided by a private chart,
of which there is no duplicate."[5] So set sail into each new
day with the expectation of discovering *something*. As you
do, you may have a "eureka" moment. If so, however, keep
in mind that streaking through your neighborhood shouting
"I've got it!" may elicit more than just looks of surprise from
your neighbors!

| 7 |

Discover Your Gold Mind

Brain cells continually produce new dendrites and receptors, grow new synapses . . . and alter the essence of the neurotransmitter soup that stimulates brain activity.

—Jean Carper[1]

We have a "gold mind" at our disposal in the form of the more than fifty neurotransmitters that surge through our brain every moment of every day. These neurotransmitters have exotic names and job descriptions and are worthy of our scrutiny. Some of the most famous are: serotonin, norepinephrine, dopamine, and GABA (gamma-aminobutyric acid).

Neurotransmitters are chemical messengers stored in tiny packets located throughout the brain and GI tract that enable neurons to communicate with one another. When a neurotransmitter is released it flashes across the junction or synapse at the end of one brain cell onto the receptor of another. Since each neuron can have multiple synapses it has the ability to communicate with literally thousands of other neurons each microsecond! This amazing ability enables us to maintain positive moods and attitudes. The health of our neurotransmitter system also affects such important functions as memory, intelligence, and even creativity.

In 2007, researchers at MIT discovered a key player in the complex chain of events controlling the release of our neurotransmitters from neuron to neuron. Tiny proteins, called complexins, are the gatekeepers. "The neurotransmitters are like racehorses. They chomp at the bit until they get the signal to dash toward the finish line. . . . Complexins are the gatekeepers that prevent the neurotransmitters from releasing prematurely."[2] Scientists hope that learning to regulate this machinery will lead to the ability to undo some of the damage from certain neurologic diseases.

Neurotransmitters are so vital to keeping traffic moving on our biochemical highway that without them our brain would instantly cease to function. Not one message could be sent or received, and the power would go out. Because these messengers are so important to *who we are*, scientists have been relentless in studying ways to protect and strengthen them. Genetics play a part, and some of us inherit lower levels of certain neurotransmitters; others have depleted amounts due to overwhelming stressful life experiences. When the makeup of our neurotransmitters is out of balance, depression and its companions take over. We feel "burned out," sad, and angry at ourselves or others. When this occurs it is imperative that we make an appointment with a trusted physician, because these days really good help is available. Antidepressants can, in a fairly short time, balance our neurotransmitter levels and improve our symptoms.

Dave's friend Forrest said, "About three years ago three unrelated events happened in succession, and this triggered my first major depression—my mother died, I turned fifty, and I quit a job I loved because I didn't see eye-to-eye with my supervisor. Over the next year, I gradually slid into the muck of despair. For the first six months I was barely functional. Then it just seemed that my energy left. I could hardly get out of bed. I felt so alone, worthless, mired in misery and emotional pain. I even prayed to die. I sensed that my marriage was suffering, and that just added to my feelings of worthlessness.

"Finally my wife, Connie, confronted me, saying, 'Something has to change. You can't go on like this. You have to get help.' Asking for help was the hardest thing I've ever done, partly due to my pride. After all I've been a Christian forty years. Shouldn't I be able to help myself? Providentially, only two days after I decided to ask for help, a depression support group was started in a local church. I'll never forget that first meeting, because when I walked in, my primary feeling was that I would rather be *anywhere* other than there. I didn't want to have to describe my struggles, but it was clear from the outset that the room was occupied by a group of special people, each with his or her own story, almost all of them a lot like my own. *So, maybe I'm not so strange*, I thought.

"From that night on, hope took root in my heart . . . hope that I might someday experience joy again."[3]

In addition to support and medication, research has also led to a series of unexpected discoveries that concluded that the type of neurotransmitters our brains make and how they travel about depends in part on what we eat. This thought would have been considered laughable before the early work of Dr. Richard Wurtman at the Massachusetts Institute of Technology in 1970. Since that time it has become accepted that the seat of our emotions, the limbic system, needs certain nutrients in order to function properly. Good fats, like Omega-3 fatty acids found in fish, can help ward off depression. A well-rounded diet that includes a reasonable amount of protein and a wide variety of whole food nutrients, including green leafy plants, is essential to maintaining brain health. Proteins are the building blocks of neurotransmitters and are crucial to balancing levels of dopamine and serotonin, for instance. It is encouraging to know that eating a healthy, varied diet helps to enhance our "gold mind" day by day.[4]

| 8 |

Dodge a Stroke

"While some risk factors cannot be controlled—such as age, gender, and family history of stroke—there are many things people can do to reduce the possibility of stroke."

—John Gullotta, M.D., Chair of AMA's
Public and Preventative Health Committee[1]

We all want to avoid a stroke. A hard look at statistics reveals the devastation of this potential killer. Stroke is the third leading cause of death in the U.S., where over 143,579 die each year. It is also a leading cause of disability. The risk of having a stroke more than doubles each decade after age fifty-five.[2] A stroke can take your life, or just ravage your *quality* of life, since it affects the way you talk, move, think, and how you eat and drink.[3] It even affects emotions and the way you can interact with those you love.

Researchers have discovered that there is a "stroke belt" stretching across the Southeastern U.S. The states involved are North Carolina, South Carolina, Georgia, Tennessee, Alabama, Mississippi, Arkansas, and Louisiana. Sadly, death rates from stroke there are a full 30-40 percent higher than in the rest of the country! A large study, called REGARDS, was begun about sixty years ago to help solve this dilemma. The investigation found that just residing in this beautiful part of the United States does not in itself mean you will suffer a stroke, but that avoiding the cultural trap of unhealthy behaviors is crucial to stroke-proofing your brain if you live there. This trap includes an unhealthy diet and smoking, among other factors. Dr. Stephen Page, one of the researchers, explains, "smoking and that whole class of unhealthy behaviors may be more common in those areas (the Southeast). They are tobacco producing states, and there are places in the South where smoking is more common, and high blood pressure and diabetes are higher. Diet and genetics can certainly play a role; genetics can interact with nutrition and change the way the genes are expressed. The 'Southern diet' of fried chicken, fried vegetables, fried potatoes, and fried everything else may contribute to the problem. Also lifestyle . . . exercise and healthy behaviors aren't as common."[4] The bottom line of this study is that you can live in the stroke belt and not be any more likely to suffer a stroke if you make an effort to *live a healthy lifestyle.*

For much of the twentieth century, little was known about the dangers of high cholesterol, lack of exercise, and even smoking, and most families were not what today we would call "health-conscious." Stroke was an all too common occurrence. Bobbie knows firsthand the devastation that comes from this crippler, because her dad suffered a stroke after open-heart surgery.

Dad was in the hospital recovering well and the family was just beginning to relax and enjoy the extra time we could spend together as we rallied around him that first week after his surgery. But then one morning as I was helping dad with his breakfast, he suddenly had difficulty chewing and seemed a little confused. Afraid that he might be having a stroke I ran to alert the nurse and she immediately paged his physician, who "happened" to be making rounds on the other side of the hall. A blood thinning medicine was immediately given as the physician diagnosed a "stroke in progress." We were devastated. Over the next few hours the family gathered and anxiously waited as dad was rushed back to surgery; this time to clear his carotid arteries. We walked the floor and prayed that the damage would be minimal and that dad would come out of surgery with his personality and function intact. We were finally called to the recovery room where dad was just waking up. As we gathered around his bed my sister quipped, "I know you are glad that is over, dad." And we were elated when he replied with a favorite phrase, "You better believe it!" However, as the days went by we realized that there was residual brain damage that would affect his quality of life. We all lost "a piece of dad" that day in the hospital and, although we were so thankful that he had retained his speech and the use of his limbs, he had forever lost his mental sharpness, the ability to play the golf game he loved, and his quick wit.

Prevention is the place to focus, so we need to learn about the risk factors and aggressively adhere to those factors that we *can* control.[5] Obviously, we can't control our gender, race, and family history. We can't control our age and present medical history. For example, if a person has had a heart attack or suffers from sleep apnea or atrial fibrillation (a condition in which the heart beats abnormally), they are at higher risk for stroke. Risk increases for everyone after age fifty-five. And recently women have edged ahead of men in number of strokes. The death rate for women from stroke is twice that of breast cancer. For those who have any of these risk factors, it is even more imperative to alter those that *can be controlled.*

Seven important risk factors are under our control, of which we have mentioned healthy diet, exercise, and not smoking. The other four are: present health conditions, taking hormones, use of illicit drugs or excessive alcohol, and obesity:

- If you have any chronic diseases such as high blood pressure, diabetes, or high cholesterol, be especially vigilant in managing them well. Carefully follow your doctor's recommendations for medication, diet, and exercise, which make a world of difference.
- Taking hormone replacement therapy (HRT) during menopause or using birth control pills can increase the risk of a blood clot.
- Illicit drug or excessive alcohol use is linked to higher incidence of stroke for both men and women.
- Obesity increases your risk of stroke, so it is critical that you work with your doctor to get your weight into a healthy range. Next time, and every time, choose the salad versus the "bloomin' onion" and the veggie medley versus the french fries. One by one, these choices add up.

A stroke is a true medical emergency, and an ambulance should be called immediately if you notice any of these three signs that can occur if a person is having a stroke:

- Face—Can the person smile? Has their mouth drooped?
- Arms—Can the person raise both arms?
- Speech—Can the person speak clearly and understand what you say?

It's tempting to leave this all up to chance, as many people do. But a 2009 study found that significant lifestyle changes can lower your stroke risk. Researchers studied four risk factors: high LDL (bad cholesterol), low HDL (good cholesterol), high triglycerides (blood fat), and high blood pressure. The study group was large—4,731 people—all of whom had suffered a recent stroke or mini stroke. Those who reached the optimum level in all four categories were 65 percent less likely to have another stroke as compared to those who did not reach optimum levels related to any of these four factors:

- LDL lower than 70
- HDL higher than 50
- Triglycerides less than 150
- Blood pressure less than 120/80[6]

This study underlines how critical it is to partner with your doctor to get your cholesterol and blood pressure into a safe range. Knowing it is possible to dodge a stroke, even if you have already experienced one, should provide a sense of hope and the determination to focus on a healthy lifestyle.

| 9 |

Don't Eat Squirrel Brains

In our family, we saw it as a prized piece of meat, and if he [Dad] shared it with you, you were pretty happy. Not that he was stingy, but there's just not much of a squirrel brain.

—Janet Norris Gates[1]

Squirrel brains are a backwoods Southern delicacy, especially in Kentucky, where the gray squirrel has been the state's official wild game animal since 1968, with an annual harvest estimated at 1.5 million. In some rural areas the predilection for this particular treat owes itself to tradition as well as to taste. According to a *New York Times* article, "Families that eat [squirrel] brains follow only certain rituals. 'Someone comes by the house with just the head of a squirrel,' Dr. Weisman said, 'and gives it to the matriarch of the family. She shaves the fur off the top of the head and fries the head whole. The skull is cracked open at the dinner table and the brains are sucked out.' It is a gift-giving ritual. The second most popular way to prepare squirrel brains is to scramble them in white gravy, he said, or to scramble them with eggs. In each case, the walnut-sized skull is cracked open and the brains are scooped out for cooking."[2]

Drs. Erick Weisman and Joseph Berger, Kentucky physicians, noted that in the four years prior to 1997, eleven cases of a human form of transmissible spongiform encephalopathy, called Creutzfeldt-Jakob disease (similar to mad cow disease), had been diagnosed in rural western Kentucky. All the patients were squirrel-brain eaters; thus, the new disease name "mad squirrel disease."[3]

Despite the findings, "Philip Lyvers, a farmer and hunter in central Kentucky whose wife simmers squirrels, head and all, with sautéed onions and peppers and serves them over rice, said 'two guys' opinions' in a medical journal won't make him change his ways. 'I know more old hunters than I know of old doctors,' Lyvers said."[4]

Eating brains or any parts of the central nervous system is somewhat risky, although in addition to squirrel brains, the brains of pigs, horses, cattle, monkeys, chickens, and goats are consumed with gusto in some parts of the world. Through October 2009, 165 people in Britain, and forty-four elsewhere, had died from mad cow disease (bovine spongiform encephalopathy-BSE).[5] Since the first outbreak of this disease, mad cows have been identified in the U.S., Canada, and Japan, and millions of cattle have been slaughtered in order to prevent the spread of the disease, which occurs through eating infected meat and bone meal. Someone joked that the result of this crisis was "the herd shot 'round the world." Others just ignore the risk, including cow brain lovers in places like Evansville, Indiana, where deep-fried cow brain sandwiches remain on the menu in some restaurants.[6]

The disease-causing agents in brains are called "prions," which are infectious proteins that cause microscopic holes in the brain. These proteins resist being broken down by the body's natural enzymes. Once infection happens, there is no treatment; the disease is uniformly fatal.[7] In the laboratory, some prions have been shown to survive up to about 250 degrees Fahrenheit, while it is estimated that the prions that cause chronic wasting disease (CWD) in deer, elk, and Shiras moose can survive to 800 degrees Fahrenheit. The latter disease has been increasing in the U.S., especially in the Rocky Mountain region, since it was discovered in 1967. Only recently has the mode of transmission been discovered; specifically, the disease is passed through infected droppings, which means that the prions may be able to survive indefinitely where they land and may come into contact with feeding animals. Also, since they are virtually indestructible in nature, they are gradually leached into the soil by rain and snow. There have been some scares, but no known transmission of CWD from animal to human by the consumption of meat. However, it is strongly recommended that the brains of harvested game be tested (state wildlife divisions offer this service free of charge), and that all wild game consumers avoid contact with or consumption of any parts of the central nervous system of these animals.

Several other meat-borne diseases can affect your brain. According to an ABC News report, Rosemary Alvarez of Phoenix thought she had a brain tumor. But on the operating table her doctor discovered something even more unsightly—a parasitic worm eating her brain. Alvarez, 37, was first referred to the Barrow Neurological Institute at St. Joseph's Hospital and Medical Center in Phoenix with balance problems, difficulty swallowing and numbness in her left arm.

An MRI scan revealed a foreign growth at her brain stem that looked just like a brain tumor to Dr. Peter Nakaji, a neurosurgeon at the Barrow Neurological Institute. "Ones like this that are down in the brain stem are hard to pick out," said Nakaji. "And she was deteriorating rather quickly, so she needed it out." Yet at a key moment during the operation to remove the fingernail-sized tumor, Nakaji, instead, found a parasite living in her brain, a tapeworm called Taenia solium, to be precise. "I was actually quite pleased," said Nakaji. "As neurosurgeons, we see a lot of bad things and have to deliver a lot of bad news." When Alvarez awoke, she heard the good news that she was tumor-free and she would make a full recovery. But she also heard the disturbing news of how the worm got there in the first place. Nakaji said someone, somewhere, had served her food that was tainted with the feces of a person infected with the pork tapeworm parasite. "It wasn't that she had poor hygiene, she was just a victim," said Nakaji.[8]

Pork tapeworm has been around for thousands of years, and millions of people have it, in their GI tract, mostly in the undeveloped world. Unless attached to feces, it cannot affect the brain. So in addition to being careful *what* you eat, be careful *where* you eat, and *who* prepares the food.

Trichinosis is another threat to your brain, as well as to your body. The 1982 Swedish biographical drama *Flight of the Eagle* (nominated for the Academy Award for Best Foreign Language Film in 1983) was based on Per Olof Sundman's novelization of the true story of S. A. Andrée's Arctic balloon expedition of 1897, an ill-fated effort to reach the North Pole in which all three expedition members perished. Andrée and companions were trying to be the first to reach the North Pole using a hydrogen balloon, but the three were never heard from again. Their bodies were discovered thirty-three years later. A detailed analysis of the evidence, including their journals, concluded that the cause of their deaths was not starvation or even freezing to death, but the ingestion of Trichinella parasites from undercooked meat from polar bears they had shot. Evidently, by the time of their deaths, the adventurers had experienced not only the typical digestive trouble, general illness, and exhaustion that comes with trichinosis, but the parasites had passed the blood-brain barrier, a rare but not unheard of result of ingesting undercooked infected meat.

As one medical report explains: "In trichinosis, inflammatory changes are brought about by the larval worms (*Trichinella spiralis*) at diverse anatomic sites, with encystation in several of the striated muscles (diaphragm, intercostals, pectoral, deltoid, biceps, gastrocnemius, etc.). Encysted larvae may remain alive in the muscle for a year. Symptoms include periorbital edema, pronounced myalgia, fatigue, precordial pain, tachycardia, hypotension, diarrhea, fever which may reach 105.8° F. Subungual splinter hemorrhages may be observed. Myocarditis may be a grave complication. Neurologic involvement may result in headache, blurred vision, photophobia, tinnitus, convulsions, delirium, coma, spastic paralysis, monoplegia, hemiplegia and polyneuritis."[9]

Trust us, these are not symptoms that anyone wants to experience, especially not arctic explorers hauling a sled over the ice after crash landing their balloon. But you can avoid trichinosis by cooking potentially infected meat (pigs, wild boar, bears—including polar bears—dogs, cats, rats, foxes, and wolves) to an internal temperature not less than 137° F, which kills the parasite. To be safe, make it 140 or even 150. To be really safe, stick to pork that you know has not been handled improperly and has been fully cooked, like a Luau Kālua pig that has been cooked all day, Hawaiian style, in an imu!

| 10 |

Don't Let Your Habits Become Addictions

Habit, if not resisted, soon becomes necessity.

—St. Augustine[1]

Most of us are well aware of the dangers of alcohol and drug addiction, as these have become rampant since the drug culture began in the 1960s and much has been researched and written about them. Through studying the brain and brain chemicals, scientists are beginning to develop a deeper understanding of how addictive and dependent behaviors start, how to treat them, and how they affect us physically and psychologically.

There is much disagreement as to what constitutes an addiction. According to Joseph Frascella, director of the division of clinical neuroscience at the National Institute on Drug

Abuse, "Addictions are repetitive behaviors in the face of negative consequences, the desire to continue doing something you know is bad for you."[2] We can become addicted, dependent, or compulsively obsessed with any activity, substance, object, or behavior that gives us pleasure.

Some researchers believe there is a similarity between *physical addiction* to substances, and *psychological dependence* involved in such activities as compulsive gambling, use of the internet, sex, shopping, and eating disorders. It is thought that these activities produce beta-endorphins in the brain, which makes the person feel "high." It is believed that if a person continues to engage in the activity to achieve this feeling of well-being and euphoria, he or she may get into an addictive cycle. This causes the individual to become physically addicted to his or her own brain chemicals, thus leading to the continuation of the behavior even when it may have serious physical, psychological, and social consequences.[3]

In looking at addictions and the brain, scientists have discovered a series of events in the brain leading up to an activity becoming a physical or psychological dependence or addiction. When neurons in the reward pathway in the brain release the neurotransmitter dopamine into brain cells, it causes pleasure or a sense of feeling good. This signal is passed to each nerve cell in the brain across a synapse. Dopamine is released into the synapse and binds to the receptors, providing a jolt of pleasure. The chemical GABA is then released, which works to prevent the receptor from being overstimulated. Addictions occur when the behavior is repeated to the point that it disrupts the normal balance of brain circuits that control rewards, memory, and cognition, leading to compulsive and addictive behavior. In other words, we become hooked not so much on the activity, but the feelings produced by the chemicals in our brains.[4]

With the use of sophisticated technology, scientists can see what goes wrong in the brain of an addict—which neurotransmitting chemicals are out of balance and what regions of the brain are affected. They are developing a more detailed understanding of how deeply and completely addiction can affect the brain, by hijacking memory-making processes and by exploiting emotions. Researchers are learning not only the short-term effects on the brain, but also the long-term effects in such areas as learning. Dopamine appears to be *the key* chemical in developing and maintaining addictions.[5]

Some of the common characteristics among addictive behaviors include: obsession with an object, activity, or substance; seeking out or engaging in the behavior even though it causes harm; compulsively engaging in the behavior; loss of control over the behavior (drinking too much, buying eight new pairs of shoes, eating a whole box of cookies, etc.); doing the behavior in secret and away from others; denial of the behavior or the extent of the behavior; and withdrawal symptoms upon cessation of the activity.[6]

As a result of increased technology and the knowledge of brain chemicals and how compulsive behaviors affect the brain, researchers over the past few years have also targeted research on the following:

Internet Addiction—The biggest issue with internet addiction is that it interrupts social relationships. Those addicted to the internet have been known to flunk out of school, repeatedly lose jobs, lose contact with friends and family, and spend hours at the computer without eating or sleeping.[7]

Sexual and Pornography Addiction—It is estimated that sixteen million people have a compulsive sexual disorder, and most are men. These addicts have become dependent on neurochemical changes in the brain during sex and are consumed by sexual thoughts.[8] Addiction to pornography usually goes along with sexual addiction. The same brain chemicals that operate with other addictions are in play when sexual and pornography addiction are involved. "The neurochemical process that happens in the brain when viewing pornography provides a high equal to that of crack cocaine."[9]

Jofizal Jannis, a doctor in Jakarta, India, reports that addiction to pornography likely harms both the structure and function of the brain, because our brain records everything it sees. Children are particularly susceptible to brain damage because their ability to filter out what they shouldn't remember is not developed until the age of thirteen. Pornography addiction in children is likely to degrade their intelligence potential.[10]

Shopping Addiction—Like other addictions, shopping can cause a high from the dopamine in the brain that switches on. The person feels good and the behavior is thus reinforced. Just as alcoholics hide their bottles, or pornography is done in secret on the internet, "shopaholics" hide their purchases. The consequences of too much shopping are obvious and many have gotten themselves into financial ruin.[11]

Gambling Addiction—Gambling addicts tend to be males from middle to upper-middle class backgrounds, often with a family history of alcoholism, depression, or compulsive gambling. Many experience a "big win" at the race track, casino, lottery, etc., and the high they feel pushes them to continue in the behavior. Their winning streak may continue for awhile as they gamble more often and bet larger amounts of money. The inevitable will happen and they start to lose. It is during this losing cycle that they deplete their own cash reserves and will often then borrow from others to cover their bets. This may eventually lead to taking illegal loans or theft to cover debts. Alienation from family and friends, job loss, physical ailments, and even suicide are often the result.[12]

The bottom line is that just about anything done in excess and that causes the pleasure centers in the brain to short-circuit with too much dopamine can become compulsive behavior that can lead to addiction. Yes, good and necessary things such as eating, sex, work, and exercise fit into this category. If you see yourself on these pages, get some help from your pastor or a counselor. Your brain is longing to be freed from the bad habits that bind you.

| 11 |

Eat Safe Fish

Eat that fish. It's brain food!
—a school lunch cook,
circa 1966

When I (Dave) was growing up, Friday was fish day in the free
school hot lunch program, for which I qualified due to my
dad being an underpaid Baptist minister in our little Vermont
town. Evidently the program's meal planners figured it was
easier to feed everybody—Protestants, Catholics, Methodists,
Episcopalians, whatever—fish on Friday, since had they not
done so, one or more of those groups might have asked for
special consideration due to their customs in those days.

So, on Fridays in school, we got some sort of fish—fish
sticks, fish cakes, cod, flounder, scrod, ocean perch, sea bass,
or whatever the government source of surplus food had to
unload that month. Strange, we never got gefilte fish.

Some of the kids seemed content to eat what was served on Fridays, perhaps because their moms had told them the same thing as my mom told me—fish is brain food. As for me, I ate my fish, and spinach, broccoli, carrots, beets, or even things of unknown origin and unknowable identity—whatever ended up on my plate day by day (with the exception of brussels sprouts). Looking back now, I wonder that none of us asked for double-blind, placebo-controlled scientific evidence to prove that eating fish was any better for our brains than a PB&J sandwich on white bread (sometimes with marshmallow worked in), or a burger and fries, with onion rings and a big Coke.

All jesting aside, I'm glad my mom and the school lunch cook made us eat our fish, because now there exists a mountain of gold standard scientific evidence that eating fish can enhance brain health. What my mom and the school cook didn't know, however, was that some fish can retain heavy metals, such as mercury, which are toxic to the brain. In general, the higher up the food chain the fish, the more likely it is to be contaminated by mercury, since the metal accumulates over time.

This was brought home in the recent past for Jim when he was practicing in Hawaii, and became an avid fan of seared tuna. After about six months of feasting on this new discovery he found that his blood mercury levels were four times normal! By switching to safer amounts and smaller fish his mercury levels returned to the normal range in just a few months and he could continue to reap all the benefits of eating fish.

Feeding your brain well may involve *learning* to like fish, with wild caught oily cold water fish being superior because of their ability to deliver Omega-3 fatty acids, which the human body needs but cannot produce on its own. Omega-3s are important throughout life, helping to maintain brain function, and may have a significant role in protecting your brain from aging. Omega-3s can be obtained from a variety of plant sources, but the most common source is fish, including wild salmon, high mountain trout, mackerel, herring, sardines, and anchovies. If you simply don't care for fish, but want some of the benefits, a variety of fish oils can be purchased locally or via the internet—but be sure that whatever you ingest is certified free of all toxins. While fish oils do not provide the protein that actually eating fish provides, this option is still healthier than ignoring your body's needs for Omega-3s and Vitamin D.

Some doctors recommend eating a half-pound of fish every week,[1] this despite the relatively disturbing 2009 report issued by the U.S. government which showed that fish in *all* of the nearly 300 streams sampled over a seven-year period contained mercury to some degree, although only about 25 percent had mercury levels exceeding what the EPA considers safe for people consuming average amounts of fish. "Mercury consumed by eating fish can damage the nervous system and cause learning disabilities in developing fetuses and young children," the report said. "The main source of mercury to most of the streams tested, according to the researchers, is emissions from coal-fired power plants. The mercury released from smokestacks here and abroad rains down into waterways, where natural processes convert it into methylmercury—a form that allows the toxin to wind its way up the food chain into fish." The report added, "Some of the highest levels [of mercury] in fish were detected in the remote blackwater streams along the coasts of the Carolinas, Georgia, Florida and Louisiana, where bacteria in surrounding forests and wetlands help in the conversion."[2]

Some fish and shellfish are contaminated with polychlorinated biphenyls or PCBs. PCBs are man-made pollutants that, although they are no longer manufactured in the U.S., have gotten into the environment, concentrating in higher levels in the food chain. PCBs and other contaminants concentrate in the fat of fish just underneath the skin. Other contaminants include dioxins and pesticides. If you catch your own fish to eat you should check on your local fish consumption advisory at the EPA web site: www.epa.gov/waterscience/fish/states.

In Pennsylvania, for example, the consumption advisory for sport fish is to not eat more than one meal of fish a week. This does not mean that you should never eat the fish you catch. It means that you should limit how much fish you eat. Fish that tend to have higher levels of mercury include shark, swordfish, king mackerel, and tilefish.[3] Fish typically low in mercury include shrimp, canned light tuna, salmon, and catfish. You can prepare fish to avoid consuming higher levels of contaminants, for example, by removing the skin and fat before you cook the fish. You can bake or broil the fish on a rack so that the fat containing the contaminants drips away from the fish.

But don't panic if you happen to eat a lot of fish one week, for example, while you are on vacation. Just cut back on fish for a few weeks afterward, and it will balance out, since your body is able to excrete mercury over time. The Environmental Defense Fund's web site (www.edf.org/seafood) has selector guides for seafood and sushi. The guides help you select a variety of fish that are high in nutrition and low in contaminants.

Studies show that aging people in some countries that consume larger amounts of fish had reduced rates of dementia and reduced losses of mental functioning. And in other countries where people eat more fish, explains the Wellness Letter from UC Berkeley, the rates of depression are lower.[4] So the bottom line is to eat the right kind of fish, one or two meals per week, because the potential health benefits outweigh the potential negatives.

For your information, there is a way to tell if the fish on your plate contains heavy metal. Lean over real close, with one ear about an inch from the fish, and listen. If you hear noise pretending to be music, then don't eat it. It's a heavy metal fish.

| 12 |

Embrace the Digital Age

Let's go surfing now, everybody's learning how.
—"Surfin' Safari," The Beach Boys (1962)

Back in the '60s, a few people surfed, though catching a wave at Malibu was then, and still is, a not-for-everyone kind of sport. Today, if you ask someone if they've been "surfing" recently, most will say yes, but they'll have in mind the much tamer waves of the internet.

In the old days (when we were in college), you had to go to the library to research anything. Today, having visited thousands of web sites while creating this series of books, we have to say that there is no doubt that while books and print articles are great, the internet has become *the* primary source of access to information on just about any topic imaginable, a lot of it free of charge.

Of all the books I (Dave) have helped create, the longest one took just over 1 megabyte of disk space. Just now I sent it to myself as an e-mail attachment, just to see how long two years' worth of wordsmithing takes to transfer from myself to myself, using AOL. Answer: 9.8 seconds. Most likely, it would have been twice as fast using my 64-bit laptop.

Today's DVD disks will hold up to 4.7 gigabytes of data. Using 1 megabyte per book as an average, you could store nearly 5,000 books on a single DVD. That number used to be impressive, when one considered the lack of access to various kinds of books in some parts of the world. As I write, I have a 64-gigabyte USB flash drive plugged into one of the ten or so USB ports built into or connected to my desktop computer. On that single flash drive, the length and width of which is about 1.5 inches by four inches, and the weight perhaps three ounces, you could store about 70,000 books.

Impressive as it may seem to be able to carry the equivalent of a library in your pocket, that size is still infinitesimal compared with the number of books that are *already* available for download via the internet. And, if Google has its way, soon you will be able to buy a vast number of books from its online library, in e-book format. All you'll need is a laptop computer with the right software, or an e-book compatible with the book service you're using, and you can order, download, store, and start to read a book of normal length in a minute or less, depending on your connection speed.

In really olden times, when we were kids, you could sign up for a "pen pal," and communicate with someone in a far-away place like France or Africa a few times a year by mail. Today, you can communicate almost instantly with anyone who is "online" and whose e-mail address you have. You can "talk" back and forth using instant messaging programs. Or better yet, you can chat in real time with anyone anywhere in the world who has an account with Skype, which also allows the addition of real-time video so, with the right equipment, you can see the person you're talking with, and they can see you—or not, depending on your preferences and the status of your makeup. As I write this sentence, there are 18,415,642 users logged on to Skype.

In less time than it took the Egyptians to build the Great Pyramid of Giza, one of the seven wonders of the ancient world, the internet, officially established in 1987, has become one of the greatest wonders this world has ever known. If you remember that Arlo Guthrie song, "You Can Get Anything You Want, at Alice's Restaurant," the internet delivers what neither the song, nor the movie that was made from the song, nor the restaurant, itself, could ever hope to deliver. Today, you can buy almost anything online. You can visit eBay, the world's largest auction "house," where a jet was sold for $4.7 million and a ghost in a jar fetched a nifty $50,922 (which the bidder never paid). You might also visit Amazon.com, the world's largest store, which started with books but now carries just about anything Alice or Arlo could want. You can buy nearly new books at Half.com for seventy-five cents plus shipping. You can buy prescription drugs online, without a prescription, from India. You can buy clothes, athletic equipment, toys, pet supplies, office supplies, a college degree, a PhD, or even get yourself ordained via the internet.

Perhaps even more importantly, since 1987 the internet has also become the world's primary social networking and "chatting" place, thanks to millions of chat rooms on any subject imaginable, and instant communication with others using today's "smart" cell phones, which have amazing capabilities, including cameras offering still and video photography, GPS guidance, and as many "apps" (applications) as one could want, with more coming. Huge networks such as Twitter,

Flickr, MySpace, Facebook, and YouTube make it possible for *anyone* with internet access, worldwide, to become aware of *anything* that is going on in the world, within seconds of the event in question having happened. For example, when U.S. Airways Flight 1549 crash landed in the Hudson River in January 2009, and all aboard survived, the *first* images broadcast from the site were captured not by news reporters dispatched to the scene, but by a cell phone camera of someone on a ferry rushing to the scene. Even before the passengers and crew were rescued, the photo was published worldwide using TwitPic, a division of Twitter. Flickr is dedicated primarily to photos and videos. MySpace and Facebook are among the largest social networking sites. Just now, when I checked, Facebook had 5.7 million users. And on YouTube, you can find video and audio of just about anything, including the Beach Boys singing "Surfin' Safari" in 1962.

According to a Wikipedia.com article on the history of the internet, "A study conducted by JupiterResearch anticipates that a 38 percent increase in the number of people with online access will mean that, by 2011, 22 percent of the Earth's population will surf the internet regularly. The report says 1.1 billion people currently enjoy regular access to the Web. For the study, JupiterResearch defined online users as people who regularly access the internet by dedicated internet access devices. Those devices do not include cell phones.

"[Since 2001] the growth of the mobile phone based internet was initially a primarily Asian phenomenon with Japan, South Korea and Taiwan all soon finding the majority of their internet users accessing by phone rather than by PC. Developing World countries followed next, with India, South Africa, Kenya, Philippines and Pakistan all reporting that the majority of their domestic internet users accessed on a mobile phone rather than on a PC.

"The European and North American use of the internet was influenced by a large installed base of personal computers, and the growth of mobile phone internet use was more gradual, but had reached national penetration levels of 20%–30% in most Western countries. In 2008 the cross-over happened, when more internet access devices were mobile phones than personal computers. In many parts of the developing world, the ratio is as much as 10 mobile phone users to one PC user on the internet."[1]

While some may detest and decry the internet, like most other things, it's not as cut and dried as some may think. Yes, like most other things, it can be used for evil. But I have no doubt that the editing and writing career and the ministry I've had over the past twenty years or so could not have happened without the internet. I have co-authored two books with someone I only met once, years before we "wrote" a word together. We created the books using e-mail and text exchanges, primarily. I've launched a print-on-demand publishing endeavor to help aspiring authors into print, with the whole process from manuscript to published book being handled totally online. And I've edited a national magazine (*Today's Christian Doctor*) for going on twenty years, from my desktop and laptop computers, whether I was in Colorado, California, Ohio, New Hampshire, Florida, or even Poland. Today, I'm writing this book in conjunction with Jim and Bobbie Dill, who are, as I write these words, en route from Hawaii to American Samoa. In the three years we've been creating this series, we've only been together in person once. With the internet, it doesn't matter where you are, or where your associates are. It only matters that you have a good computer and software, and a good connection.

In retrospect, I feel like all these years of writing, editing, and surfing, since I got my first computer in about 1984, have kept my mind as sharp as it can be, at the "middle age" of sixty. One thing is for sure; thanks to computers and the internet, I can't remember being bored, nor can I imagine what some of my contemporaries from our college class of 1970 are longing for—retirement. It's a wonderful age in which to be alive, and the internet is part of the reason.

Researchers are finding that using the internet can significantly engage brain activity in middle-aged and older adults, with improvements shown right from the start. Using high-tech non-invasive functional magnetic resonance imaging (fMRI) scans, UCLA scientists were able to track brain activity by measuring the level of blood flow in the brain during cognitive tasks. They reported that "searching the internet triggers key centers in the brain that control decision-making and complex reasoning. The findings demonstrate that Web search activity may help stimulate and possibly improve brain function.

" 'The study results are encouraging, that emerging computerized technologies may have physiological effects and potential benefits for middle-aged and older adults,' said principal investigator Dr. Gary Small, a professor at the Semel Institute for Neuroscience and Human Behavior at UCLA who holds UCLA's Parlow-Solomon Chair on Aging. 'internet searching engages complicated brain activity, which may help exercise and improve brain function.'

"Small noted that pursuing activities that keep the mind engaged may help preserve brain health and cognitive ability. Traditionally, these include games such as crossword puzzles, but with the advent of technology, scientists are beginning to assess the influence of computer use—including the internet."[2]

My parents are both in their eighties. One of their regular activities is to play the word games Pathword and Scramble, both of which they access through Facebook. They both enjoy competing with other family members and friends to see who can get the highest score in these games. While I haven't joined that good-natured word fray yet, I think I'll have to do so, someday, if only to demonstrate that publishing a million-plus words does not make one a word-meister.

Yes, there are dangers in surfing, whether in Malibu or on the internet. But some very good times can be had, whether mastering the perfect pipeline wave, or coming up with the all-time highest Pathword score of anyone you know. It's all relative in the end. But our suggestion is that in the best interest of keeping your mind sharp, you become as computer savvy as you can become, acquire the best equipment you can afford, and then learn to use it wisely and well, including how to safely and productively surf the Net, which will keep your synapses firing instead of retiring.

| 13 |

Enjoy Sports

Games lubricate the body and the mind.

—Benjamin Franklin[1]

You've had a rough week and all you want to do on the weekend is veg out in front of the TV with your favorite snacks and watch your favorite sports shows. If anyone asked you what your favorite sport is, you might just say, "yes," because sometimes it really doesn't matter as long as you can lose yourself in the game, any game. Ladies, you're probably thinking, *That sounds just like my husband!* But according to a study done by Scarborough Sports Marketing, over the last twenty years women have become more passionate about professional sports. Also, according to *Media Life* magazine, by 2002 one third of the viewers of Monday Night Football were women.[2] By the 2007–08 racing season, 37.6 percent of NASCAR fans were women. The lure for women is the same as for men: exciting games and the opportunity to participate by proxy. So the next time you're at the ballpark or stadium, check it out—much of the crowd consists of women. Watching and participating in sports is no longer just a "guy thing," which in some cases could be a marriage-saver.

It is estimated that 69 percent of the American people watch sports. A Harris Interactive Poll published in 2008 reported that football is America's favorite sport, followed by baseball, college football, and auto racing.[3] With the popularity of the internet, fans can follow their favorite sport(s) online. Approximately thirty million people play fantasy sports in the U.S.

Participating in sports is good for you. Do you like to walk? How about beefing it up and starting to train for a half or full marathon? Running isn't a requirement—many people choose to walk the course. Walking improves your ability to make decisions, solve problems, and to focus. It's also a great stress buster and you'll sleep better at night. Aerobic activities release hormones, such as adrenaline and endorphins. These are good for your nervous system, boosting your mood, relieving pain, and creating a sense of well-being. Also, if you train with a friend, you're more likely to keep going, and the social connection is also good for your mental functioning.[4]

Let's say you're actively engaged in some kind of physical activity or sport, but still enjoy following your favorite team(s) on TV. Maybe it's the day of the big game and you invite some friends over to watch. You enjoy discussing the play-by-play, talking the language of the game, and, if it's football, being an armchair quarterback. According to research conducted by the University of Chicago, you can improve brain functioning *both by participating in and watching sports.* "Being an athlete or merely a fan improves language skills when it comes to discussing their sport because parts of the brain usually involved in playing sports are instead used to understand sport language."[5]

"For the study, researchers asked 12 professional and intercollegiate hockey players, eight fans and nine individuals who had never watched a game to listen to sentences about hockey players, such as shooting, making saves and being engaged in the game. They also listened to sentences about everyday activities, such as ringing doorbells and pushing brooms across the floor. While the subjects listened to the sentences, their brains were scanned using MRI, which allows one to infer the areas of the brain most active during language listening." After hearing the sentences, the subjects were given tests which would gauge their understanding of those sentences. Most subjects understood the language about everyday activities, and it's reasonable that hockey players and fans understood hockey-related language better than the novices.[6]

The results showed "that a region of the brain usually associated with planning and controlling actions is activated when players and fans listen to conversations about their sport. The brain boost helps athletes' and fans' understanding of information about their sport and the language connected with it. Playing sports, or even just watching, builds a stronger understanding of language. Brain areas usually used to act become highly involved in language understanding. There is a change in the neural networks that support comprehension in incorporating areas active in performing sports skills."[7]

Sue loves to watch football. For her, there is nothing more exciting than watching her favorite teams duke it out on a Sunday afternoon in the fall. Church in the morning and football in the afternoon. She prints out the NFL schedule in August and keeps track of how "her teams" are doing throughout the season. It's especially exciting when one of her favorite teams is in the playoffs. She enjoys talking about the games with friends and co-workers and can hold her own in these conversations. Now, she admits that she doesn't know a blitz from a quarterback option, but she can follow the ball down the field, know about downs, field goals and touchdowns, and so on. She can identify the quarterback, but isn't so sure about the rest of the players. She sometimes wonders: *Is he a running back, fullback, or some other kind of back? It really doesn't matter, does it? It's the excitement of the game that has me hooked.*

Evidently, according to the research, it's okay to be hooked on watching your favorite sports, in moderation of course. Those small pleasures can translate into good health for your brain. So, grab a healthy snack, curl up on the couch, and watch that game. Engage yourself with the strategies and execution of various calls. Try to understand clock management, if it applies. Learn as many of the rules as your brain will tolerate. Turn the sound off from time to time, and see how many of the signals given by the officials you can understand without hearing what is said. Play the game in your mind as it progresses. While your favorite team may not win every game, it's still fun and it can be healthy for the functioning of your brain.

| 14 |

Equip Your Brain by Exercising Your Heart

A strong link was found between physical activity and brain health . . . older people who exercise are less likely to experience cognitive decline.

—Panel made up of three institutes of the National Institute of Health[1]

This is cause for celebration! Research shows that we are not total victims of our genes and that lifestyle, especially physical exercise, will help equip our brains for the journey before us. We have heard again and again that exercise will control cardiovascular risk factors and give new life to almost every organ system in our body. Now we can add brain health to the list.

The connection between cardiovascular exercise and brain function has been studied by many teams who have concluded that moderate exercise triggers a release of neurotropins in the hippocampus or memory area of the brain. Neurotropins are hard workers that promote growth and repair of neural tissue. Neurotropins have been studied in animals and are clearly shown to counteract the ravages of diseases affecting memory. Studies are underway to determine if physical exercise could prevent symptoms for years in people who are at genetic risk for Alzheimer's disease.[2]

You may be thinking, *I am over fifty and have not exercised a day in my life. Is it too late to start?* Doctors assure us that it is never too late to begin to take advantage of all the benefits exercise has to offer. Not only will you delay mental decline, you will also likely notice an improvement in mood and more control over your response to stress.

A visit to your doctor is a good first step and he/she will guide you on your way to a good exercise regime. You may be relieved to know that research has proven, when it comes to exercise and the brain, that harder is not necessarily better. Moderate exercise is the level that has been shown to produce the most positive brain results. In fact, biologist Andrew Naylor showed in animal studies that over-exercising is not good for the brain. While new stem cells were produced after nine days of exercising with a third of them remaining to become functioning nerve cells, over-exercising resulted in only half as many new hippocampal nerve cells as in the animals that did not exercise at all. The theory is that if too much of the body's own morphine (endorphin) and stress hormones are produced, it actually retards the brain's ability to make new brain cells. Doctors will usually recommend thirty- to forty-five-minute sessions of moderate exercise four or five days a week for most people at 60 percent of your maximum pulse rate, unless of course you happen to be an elite athlete, in which case the target pulse rate will be higher.[3]

Dr. Debbye T. Bell, a broadcast journalist, recently reported on CBS's *The Early Show* that exercise does in fact make you smarter. Here is some of what she had to say as she interviewed and quoted several educators and researchers in the field:

> One school in Illinois has developed a program that gets kids moving and learning. Although it may appear that these kids are working out, they are actually trying to adjust their brain chemistry to maximize their ability to learn.
>
> "We're putting kids in P.E. class prior to classes that they struggle in and what we're doing is we're finding great, great results," said Paul Zientarski, who helps run a learning readiness program at Naperville Central High School in Illinois. The program was started in response to research showing a link between exercise and increased brain function. He says that he has seen the results. "Kids who took P.E. before they took the math class had double the improvement of kids who had P.E. afterward," Zientarski explained.
>
> "Exercise optimizes the brain and the person for learning. It creates the right environment for all of our 100 billion nerve cells up there," says Dr. John Ratey, a professor of psychiatry at the Harvard Medical School and the author of *Spark*, a book that examines how our brains change when we exercise. "It produces these growth factors . . . and I call it miracle grow for the brain or brain fertilizer which helps the brain cells stay alive, live longer and it helps the learning process," Ratey said. . . .
>
> Naperville Central High School has embraced the idea that working out helps a child learn. There you can find exercise equipment in some classrooms.
>
> "Their bodies are moving and their brains are thinking and they're engaged—not sitting still trying to memorize something," says Maxyne Kozil, a reading teacher, who believes that kids learn best when they're moving. An example of this is having a student work on her vocabulary while standing on balance boards. "They say having to balance actually helps them to concentrate even better," Kozil said.

In their math classes students rarely zone out because every so often they take a "brain break . . . interactive games that get kids up and out of their seats. . . .

What's ironic is that some schools have cut back on P.E. in favor of academics when actually research is showing that physical exercise is exactly what kids need in order to excel.[4]

We (Bobbie and Jim) had a great opportunity to observe this up close when we had the unexpected pleasure of being offered a temporary hospital assignment very close to our son and granddaughter's hometown. Spending three months immersed in our granddaughter Kendal's world brought new insights and immeasurable joy to every day! We noticed right away as we picked her up from school that every fiber in her eight-year-old body was yearning to run and play, so we got to be kids again as we climbed monkey bars and played soccer and hide-and-seek! We did decline on the cartwheels and rolling down hills! After this kind of exercise, Kendal was ready to settle into her favorite place to do homework while Bobbie started dinner. We noticed how quickly she breezed through the math and reading, happily perched, of all places, on top of the kitchen counter! From her lofty seat she could stretch or climb up and down a few times when a math problem needed some extra thought and we could cheer her on as she finished each page. It took all the "work" out of making sure all the homework got done. And then she could even teach us some of her newly learned science facts.

We have taken this lesson from Kendal to heart and try to intersperse as much physical exercise into our day as possible by taking even short breaks from the intensity of our work and trying whenever possible to make our brain-friendly exercise sessions fun. In fact, I think I will take a spin around the block right now!

| 15 |

Feed Your Neurons Well

Americans get more of their antioxidants from coffee than any other dietary source.

—Joe Vinson, PhD[1]

Feeding your brain well begins in childhood, and continues throughout life. Those fortunate to have a parent who insisted on the consumption of healthy foods usually develop lifelong habits that enhance health and thwart disease. Those who are not so fortunate may develop childhood eating habits that are difficult to change.

In his conclusion to a scientific study, "Micronutrients and Alzheimer's Disease," author Hannes B. Staehelin wrote, "Of potentially far-reaching consequences is the concept that nutritional conditions in early life may programme metabolic functions, leading over time to an increasing imbalance and thus favouring the emergence of disease states. A macronutrient and micronutrient intake that has preventive effects against CVD [cardiovascular disease] is most likely also to be effective against neurodegenerative disorders."[2]

Translation: The protection of the health of one's brain is a lifelong endeavor, and eating habits formed in one's youth often continue throughout one's entire life.

So, if you're a parent of growing children, make it your mission to feed them as well as possible, and thus "program" their preferences for life.[3] But even if you're middle-aged or older, and you've been living on fast food and junk food and processed food with all the trans fats, sugars, salts, additives, and preservatives that have helped them sell since about 1950, it's never too late to give your body a chance to repair itself, cell by cell—and thankfully, studies are showing that such repair can even occur in the brain.

Consuming a wide variety of whole foods—fruits, vegetables, grains, nuts and berries—regularly is the most brain-friendly approach. A summary of research published in the August 2009 issue of *Journal of Alzheimer's Disease* states: "Researchers have investigated the relationship between fruit and vegetable intake, plasma antioxidant micronutrient status and cognitive performance in healthy subjects aged 45 to 102 years. The study results . . . indicate higher cognitive performance in individuals with high daily intake of fruits and vegetables. Subjects with a high daily intake (about 400 g) of fruits and vegetables had higher antioxidant levels, lower indicators of free radical-induced damage against lipids as well as better cognitive performance compared to healthy subjects of any age consuming low amounts (<100 g/day) of fruits and vegetables. Modification of nutritional habits aimed at increasing intake of fruits and vegetables, therefore, should be encouraged to lower the prevalence of cognitive impairment."[4]

Over the past decade or so, science has been uncovering evidence that the micronutrients in whole foods help fight "oxidative stress," increasingly being blamed for contributing to degenerative diseases including those of the heart and brain. Today, entire antioxidant supplement empires sell wonder products from açaí berries to super-chocolate. But did you know that their claims are built on a theory that is only about a half-century old?

According to Wikipedia.com, "The free radical theory of aging was conceived by Denham Harman in the 1950s, when prevailing scientific opinion held that free radicals were too unstable to exist in biological systems, and before anybody had invoked free radicals as a cause of degenerative diseases."[5] Here's just another example of how yesterday's unreasonable theory becomes tomorrow's maxim. In fact, one online document describing "Power Foods: Doctors' Top Choices for Antioxidant Rich Foods," begins with this sentence: "It's common knowledge that antioxidants protect us from dangerous substances called free radicals that can lead to many chronic diseases. Science touts antioxidants and their role in everything from preventing cancer and heart disease to boosting the immune system and slowing the aging process."[6]

Food for thought: below is a list of antioxidants and the foods that can best provide them.

Beta-carotene: apricots, cantaloupe, carrots, mangos, pumpkin, sweet potatoes, and some green leafy vegetables including collard greens, kale, and spinach. (These three leafy vegetables also contain **Lutein**, essential to eye health.)

Lycopene: apricots, blood oranges, guava, papaya, pink grapefruit, tomatoes, watermelon.

Vitamin A: carrots, egg yolks, liver, milk, mozzarella cheese.

Vitamin C: fruits and vegetables, as well as cereals, beef, poultry, and fish.

Vitamin E: almonds, broccoli, mangos, nuts.

Other whole foods worth including in your brain-healthy diet include: alfalfa sprouts, beets, blackberries, blueberries (antioxidant king of the non-exotic berries), brussels sprouts, cherries, corn, eggplant, onions, oranges, plums, pomegranates, prunes, raisins, raspberries, red bell peppers, red grapes, strawberries, and unprocessed whole grains.

In terms of this whole antioxidant issue, however, one word of caution might be worth a mound of money to you. Antioxidant values (ORAC–Oxygen Radical Absorbance Capacity) are determined in a laboratory (i.e., in a test tube), and thus far no one has demonstrated that dosing or even mega dosing on manufactured sources of antioxidants enhances health or prevents disease in real, live people.

By contrast, there is overwhelming evidence that consuming a wide variety of whole foods regularly does enhance health and help prevent disease, in general, and in relation to our focus in this book, in the brain in particular. This is why we recommend that, instead of ingesting various products without knowing whether they may help or harm you, strive to fill in the gaps in your brain-health-oriented diet with real food, preferably in as close to its natural state as possible.

In general, what's good for your heart is good for your brain, because both depend on good blood flow. That's one reason why the Alzheimer's Association and the American Heart Association, along with its American Stroke Association division, launched a new public awareness program to help African-Americans manage their heart and brain health (African-Americans are at greater risk than Caucasians for developing diabetes, Alzheimer's, vascular dementia, and stroke) in February 2009. The program is called "What's good for your heart is good for your brain."[7]

That being said, since we know that for some people making significant dietary changes, especially all at once, may seem either too difficult or too distasteful, we suggest considering augmenting with food concentrates made from whole, ripe, raw fruits, vegetables, and grains.[8] Even small changes add up over time, and since developing diseases can be arrested if you will take the issue seriously enough to do more than pop some more man-made, artificial supplements, a change in time could save you nine.

Dan was raised on Southern cooking and learned early to love biscuits, fried chicken, and pecan pie! He happily feasted on his favorite foods all through high school and college with no ill effects at all. However, once he had a "real job" and spent long hours at a desk dealing with stressful issues, he slowly began to gain weight. Exercise had become a thing of the past so he tried to add in running several times a week, convinced that would solve everything. But as his weight continued to climb along with his blood pressure he knew he had to bite the dreaded bullet of dietary change. His wife was concerned enough to put time into changing his favorite recipes into low-fat varieties and began slowly adding more fruits, veggies, and whole grains into their meal plan. In addition he began taking whole food concentrates recommended by a friend. To his total surprise Dan loved the new way of eating, felt fuller after meals, and best of all began losing weight. An added benefit was the normalizing of his blood pressure, which he knew would go a long way toward preventing a heart attack like the one that took his father's life at a young age. In 2009, he and his wife celebrated five years and counting of improved health, without so much as a cold since biting the diet-change bullet!

| 16 |

Get Off the Couch

Because I only have got one brain to rot I'm gonna spend my
life watching television a lot.

—From "Couch Potato" by Weird Al Yankovic

You've heard the term "couch potato," and maybe you are
one, but do you know the phrase's origination? According
to Answers.com, "Very few words have a birthday so precise,
and so precisely known, as *couch potato*. It was on July 15,
1976, we are told, that *couch potato* came into being, uttered
by Tom Iacino of Pasadena, California, during a telephone
conversation. He was a member of a Southern California
group humorously opposing the fads of exercise and healthy
diet in favor of vegetating before the TV and eating junk food
(1973). Because their lives centered on television—the boob
tube (1966)—they called themselves *boob tubers*. Iacino ap-
parently took the brilliant next step and substituted *potato*

as a synonym for *tuber*. Thinking of where that potato sits to watch the tube, he came up with *couch potato*." This history is important because, as the explanation adds, ". . . when the new phrase reached the ears of Robert Armstrong, another member of the boob tubers, he drew a cartoon of a potato on a couch, formed a club called the Couch Potatoes, registered the trademark and began merchandising Couch Potato paraphernalia, from T-shirts to dolls. He published a newsletter called *The Tuber's Voice: The Couch Potato Newsletter* and a book, *Dr. Spudd's Etiquette for the Couch Potato*.[1]

Quite often, couch potatoes are stereotyped as overweight, slovenly men sitting around in their underwear watching a variety of events on TV, downing potato chips and other trans-fat-laden snack foods with the help of a steady supply of beer.

The term entered the Oxford English Dictionary in 1993 and is so well known in the UK that a plan of the Prime Minister's Strategy Unit tied attempts "to combat the couch potato culture" to "[improving the UK's] international sporting performance."[2] Athletic performance aside, perhaps more important to the general population is the impact of the couch potato culture on brain performance.

In her article "Is Your Brain a Couch Potato?" San Francisco internist and columnist "Doc Gurley" writes, "our brain is not static. As we age, the rule of 'use it or lose it' becomes all important to your brain—but improvements have been documented at every age, and even after injury. Brains crave novel, challenging 'out of your comfort zone' activities to thrive."[3]

With recent advancements in non-invasive technology, the new field of "brain fitness" has burst into the everyday parlance of the U.S. population, and along with it a burgeoning collection of products and programs, many of them making a killing without much, if any, verifiable research to back up their claims. For example, one program states, "[Our program] uses a scientifically-proven brain training exercise to increase mental focus, memory, and problem-solving ability by 40% in less than 20 days. [Our program] produces rapid, dramatic, and lasting benefits, guaranteed."[4] What this claim doesn't mention is that the data cited as evidence that this particular program works was not collected through the study of this program itself, but through the study of a similar program. This is referred to as "borrowed research" as opposed to "primary research." Borrowed research is considered anecdotal and unreliable, from a scientific perspective.[5]

For any such claims to be valid, they must be substantiated by the gold standard of scientific inquiry (double-blind, placebo-controlled, randomized studies). As of this writing, the only book we know of that actually evaluates the wide variety of brain training programs with this gold standard in view is *The SharpBrains Guide to Brain Fitness* by Alvaro Fernandez and Dr. Elkhonon Goldberg (2009). "Brain fitness," the authors write, "is our brain's ability to readily create additional connections between neurons, and even to promote new neurons in certain parts of the brain. Research in neuropsychology and neuroscience shows that vigorous mental activity can lead to good brain fitness, which in turn, translates into a sharper memory, faster processing of information, better attention, and other improved cognitive skills.

"In general, brain fitness products are geared to change the trajectory of the life curve so that younger minds improve their peaks (or reach them faster) and older people do not experience such a loss of various cognitive abilities, like mental flexibility, working memory, and others.

"If the brain is flexible and molded through experience, the question is, 'What tools can help provide the right kind of experience to help refine our brains, from a structural and functional point of view?' The goal of this guide is precisely to help you answer that question."[6] Later in the book, the authors list their top twenty-one picks of brain training software, organized by purpose, including eight brain maintenance products, eight targeted brain workout products, and five stress management products, with only two of the latter having "medium-high" scores for "clinical validation." In other words, the scientific jury is still out regarding the claims made in relation to such products, although their claims seems consistent with relatively new findings that a wide variety of creative engagements can stimulate the production of new neurons as long as we live.

Why not get off that couch and engage those neurons, one way or another? You don't even need to spend a bunch of money on software or programs, though such an investment might prove worthwhile. Instead why not take a walk (exercise), during which you might stop and share a nutritious picnic lunch (nutrition) with a friend (social connection), while discussing one of the most recent books (cognition) you've both read. Better yet, if you believe, as we do, that brain health also has spiritual components, center the discussion on a book with mutual spiritual significance and perhaps even add in a little prayer as you go (stress reduction and connection with God). By making choices like that day by day, year after year, your brain won't "rot," as Al Yankovic says, but it will remain sharp and fit until you don't need it anymore.

| 17 |

Go to Church

Tell me the story often, for I forget so soon; the early dew of morning has passed away at noon.

—Hymn lyrics by A. Katherine Hankey[1]

Perhaps you've wondered why so many older folks attend church so regularly. Is it a social issue—to be with other people and thus counter their feelings of loneliness or isolation? Is it a salvation issue—a way to try to earn divine credits with the One they're likely to meet sooner than later? A psychological issue—to receive encouragement, hope, and inner peace? A way to insure a church burial when the time comes? A way to feel better about themselves, at least for awhile? Or is it to strengthen their faith as well as their minds? Faith, yes, most likely, but minds? Can church attendance strengthen the mind?

Research indicates that it can, slowing cognitive decline in the healthy and further decline in those who already have Alzheimer's disease. In a *Southern Medical Journal* article titled "Religion, Spirituality, and Healthy Cognitive Aging," Terrance D. Hill, PhD, wrote, "Results showed that religious attendance, not religious identity, was associated with a reduction in the odds of cognitive dysfunction over time. Compared with those who attended religious services less than once per week, those who attended services once per week or more exhibited a 36% reduction in the odds of cognitive dysfunction over 3 years."[2]

In the same article, Dr. Hill added, "Results showed that higher levels of religiosity and religious practice were associated with slower rates of cognitive decline in Alzheimer's patients. The researchers concluded that spirituality and religious practices may delay the progression of Alzheimer's disease."[3]

Although no one knows for sure the mechanism that produces these positive results, they are consistent with other data we've shared in this series (*70 Ways to Beat 70*) about the longevity benefits of church attendance and the active pursuit of personal faith by other methods. Our own theory is that the whole experience of church attendance—including the social, psychological, and spiritual connections that occur during worship—may strengthen the biological connections known as synapses in the brain.

For example, one of our friends whom we'll call Don, is sixty. When he attends church, at a church similar to that of his youth, his connections to his lifelong faith are renewed, along with his sense of hope and even optimism that comes when one rests in the sovereignty of God during difficult times. "My dad was a Baptist minister," Don says, "so we were in church whenever the doors were open. Week after week, year after year, like the changing seasons, we heard the Scriptures read from the 'Authorized Version,' and we sang our way through the Baptist hymnal. Since neither of these has changed much in a half-century, when I attend church now, I can still sing most of those hymns, from memory, and recite a lot of the Scripture, too. Even some of the sermons seem familiar, though deliveries and personalities vary from preacher to preacher. In any case, at the end of many Sunday morning services, I feel like I've been 'home again,' in some way reconnected with what is not just familiar, but really real. Yes, sometimes I am reminded of my shortcomings, but that makes the grace of God even more special. I believe all these things clear my mind and help me focus better on what is really important in the week to come."

While this whole arena of research—the impact of faith on health—is relatively new, and there is some question about how much can or should be made of the easiest to measure variable, church attendance, it is clear that practicing one's faith, including attending church regularly, is health-enhancing. It may even help you keep your mind longer than some of your non-church-attending peers.

Other areas of investigation may show similar results from less public "church" attendance, including devotional reading or participation in small study groups. While these would be harder to quantify scientifically than discovering how often a person attends public services, there is enough evidence to show that reading can significantly reduce stress, so spiritual activities involving reading seem logical candidates for improving one's brain health.

New research by consultancy Mindlab International at the University of Sussex says:

> Reading works better and faster than other methods to calm frazzled nerves such as listening to music, going for a walk

or settling down with a cup of tea. Psychologists believe this is because the human mind has to concentrate on reading and the distraction of being taken into a literary world eases the tensions in muscles and the heart. The volunteers were monitored and their stress levels and heart rate were increased through a range of tests and exercises before they were then tested with a variety of traditional methods of relaxation. Reading worked best, reducing stress levels by 68 percent, said cognitive neuropsychologist Dr. David Lewis. Subjects only needed to read, silently, for six minutes to slow down the heart rate and ease tension in the muscles, he found. In fact it got subjects to stress levels lower than before they started.[4]

When you add in group discussion of what one has found during one's devotional reading over the past week, the social dimension kicks in again, in addition to the stimulation of your mind through sharing your own thoughts and listening to others express theirs. This is one modern way to accomplish what the Apostle Paul instructed his own disciple, Timothy, to do; specifically, to stir up the gift of God that was in him (most likely a reference to his faith, which had been passed on to him by his mother and grandmother), "For God hath not given us the spirit of fear; but of power, and of love, and of a sound mind" (2 Tim. 1:7 KJV). In small groups, sometimes called "house churches," all around the world, believers are stirring up each other's faith, thus increasing the strength of their beliefs, their love for one another, and the serious-mindedness that comes from viewing things from an eternal versus a temporal perspective.

So, however you can accomplish it, it surely makes sense to hear some part of "the old, old story" on a regular basis. And it also seems reasonable to do all we can to help our aging friends or relatives participate with us as often as possible. After all, the spiritual needs of your mother or grandmother have not diminished with aging, and their cognitive abilities may benefit from attending "church" with you, more than most people can imagine. For the Apostle Paul put no age limit on his suggestion that you can "be renewed in the spirit of your mind, and put on the new self, which in the likeness of God has been created in righteousness and holiness of the truth" (Eph. 4:23–24 NASB).

| 18 |

Improve Your Thinking Day by Day

As [a man] thinketh in his heart, so is he.
—Proverbs 23:7 KJV

Most of us want to be able to continually improve our thinking skills. The ability to think clearly, intelligently, and rapidly
is one of our greatest resources and helps us to live a successful, abundant life. We were first allowed glimpses into the
miraculous human brain during the 1990s with the invention
of advanced brain scanning techniques. This knowledge has
overturned much of our prior understanding about the way
we humans think. It is now accepted as fact that every brain
is unique, reflecting all our previous experience and education. In other words, we each have the opportunity to build
a better brain, day by day.

To build the best brain possible, we need to think like
the coach of a football team, since there are eleven ways of

thinking. As we strengthen the neuron pathways between areas of our brain, we increase our IQ. All of these thinking abilities are involved in our everyday decisions and actions, which often engage several areas of our brain at once. This neurological workout continually forges new pathways and strengthens old ones.

The thinking team players are as follows (in order from basic to complex):

Basic Level Thinking
Visual
Numerical
Recollective
Empathetic
Verbal
Predictive
Ethical
Creative
Critical
Reflective
Applied
Higher Order Thinking[1]

Activities that work these different areas of our brain are known as metacognitive activities and actually strengthen our "thinking cap," the frontal cerebral cortex or learning center. When we engage in brain-jogging activities our frontal cerebral cortex is actually thickened, much the same way working with weights will strengthen arm muscles. Our amazing brain has an automatic pilot gear (the one we use while driving home engrossed in our music or while sleeping at night) but the metacognitive thinking powerhouse must be *requested*. For instance, when we consider why we acted in a certain way, we are using *reflective thinking* skills that pull us from the past, through the present, and propel us into the future. Weakened reflective thinking can cripple our problem-solving abilities.

Professor Michael Shayer at King's College in London reported in 2006, after following 10,000 children for fifteen years, that some of the cognitive abilities of eleven- and twelve-year-olds had deteriorated on the average of two to three years compared to fifteen years earlier. The opposite was expected. Shayer speculated that the decline was because many learning activities important in elementary and secondary schools had fallen by the wayside. Art, music, and physical education had been cut from curriculums. He also suggested that creative thinking had, in too many cases, been replaced by overuse of technology (TV, video games, and calculators).[2]

Clear scientific thinking so desperately needed during those challenging academic years requires creative thinking, dependent upon a well-functioning brain. You might make a case that "Use it or lose it" applies here. For instance, *numerical thinking* enhances logic and reasoning, while improving IQ and creating extra cognitive reserve. Such a reserve is a great nest egg that can be recruited if disease or brain injury strikes in the future.

The story of Bob Woodruff's horrific traumatic brain injury (TBI) and incredible recovery has brought hope to many. This gifted reporter suffered devastating injury while covering the war in Iraq in 2006. His book, *In An Instant: A Family's Journey of Love And Healing*, documents his experience of loss and recovery. After thirty-seven days in a coma and numerous brain surgeries, Bob emerged to begin his arduous and lengthy rehab process. Bob's wife, Lee, related some of

101

his journey in a newspaper interview. "The thing I would like to say is that rehab is a long process. Doctors told me that Bob, despite the severity of his injuries, had better chances to recover than other victims, because of the reserve of neurons and connections he had built thanks to an intellectually stimulating and diverse life, including living in China for several years and traveling to dozens of countries, having worked as a lawyer and as a journalist, and his overall curiosity and desire to learn. It seems that more and more research shows how people who are mentally active throughout their lives, either through their jobs, or doing puzzles or Sudoku are, of course up to a point, better prepared to deal with problems such as traumatic brain injury. Bob had six months of structured cognitive therapy focused on speech and language areas because that was the part of his brain that had been most damaged. The therapist identified the main tasks for him to work on in a challenging, yet familiar way, usually asking Bob, for example, to read the *New York Times*, then try to remember what he had read, and write a short essay on his thoughts and impressions.

"I am amazed to watch in real time now even today, how he gets better and better. To give you an example of his motivation to recover, he recently took on Chinese lessons to see if working on that also helped him."[3]

Bob's experience has benefited military personnel and civilians afflicted with TBI and is a great incentive for all of us to build our God-given thinking skills day by day.

Dave's son, Christopher, to whom he dedicated his bestselling book *If God is So Good, Why Do I Hurt So Bad?*, is another example of the degree to which a brain injury can be overcome with courage, patience, and persistence. Christopher could read *The New York Times* by the time he was three, due in part to his interaction with the word games and other games available via the recently introduced Commodore 64. But when he was six, about to go to first grade, he experienced a metabolic brain injury (like the one that had taken the life of his older brother), as a result of which he temporarily lost all the functions controlled by the areas of his brain that were affected—speech, movement, control of bodily functions. But he still knew how to play the Commodore 64, and refused to give up, and thanks to the dogged determination of his mother, he gradually recovered to the point where he could play that game again, using a magic marker taped in his hand as a joystick. Later, he was able to get back into school, graduate high school with his own peers, and then go to college and graduate, as well. "Sometimes when I think of giving up," Dave says, "I think of Chris and all he has overcome. While none of us will ever know why our family is affected by this genetic deficiency, we do know that Chris accomplished more in a few years than just about anyone we know because he never gave up, but instead recaptured what he could and built on that. I'm still proud of him, and always will be."

| 19 |

Keep Your Nose Clean

How sense-luscious the world is.

—Diane Ackerman[1]

When you think of noses, *who* comes to mind? Cyrano de Bergerac, De Gaulle, or Pinocchio, perhaps. But how about Mehmet Ozyurek of Turkey, whose nose is longest in the world, at 4.5 inches?

When you think of noses, *what* comes to mind? Nose hair, nose warts, sneezes, snorts, runny noses, sniffling noses, blowing noses, itchy noses, nose picking, nose wrinkling, or laying a finger aside one's nose, as with Santa in the famous poem, or with others, worldwide, who use this gesture to show that they share with you some secret that must remain that way.

Or maybe you think of nose jokes like, "Your nose is so big, the only date you can get is with an anteater." Or, "I've got it all backward today. My nose is running and my feet smell."

Whoever or whatever comes to mind, your nose is no joke, and keeping it "clean" is important to the health of your body, including your brain. We breathe about 23,000 times a day, often with our mouth closed. The healthier your nose, the better your oxygenation. Beyond that, a healthy nose is crucial to your sensory enjoyment of food, flowers, and perfume, among many other things.

As Diane Ackerman wrote, "Nothing is more memorable than a smell. One scent can be unexpected, momentary and fleeting, yet conjure up a childhood summer beside a lake in the mountains; another, a moonlit beach; a third, a family dinner of pot roast and sweet potatoes during a myrtle-mad August in a Midwestern town. Smells detonate softly in our memory like poignant land mines hidden under the weedy mass of years. Hit a tripwire of smell and memories explode all at once. A complex vision leaps out of the undergrowth."[2]

It is fairly common for people to experience a loss of smell in life, temporarily. This could be from a sinus problem, a cold, or allergies. If you've ever noticed a diminished sense of taste, you were really experiencing a loss of smell. When you eat and drink, most of what you sense is due to aroma rather than taste. You can differentiate four basic tastes (sweet, salty, sour, and bitter) but you can smell a large number of different odors. When you chew and swallow food, odors in your mouth are released to travel to your nose through a back passageway, enhancing your sense of taste.

Anosmia is the loss of the sense of smell. While it has many causes, exposure to toxic chemicals, allergies, and infections can bring it on. The olfactory bulb lies near the base of your brain at the top of your nose, between your eyes. The olfactory bulb can be damaged, or the olfactory nerve that carries the messages to your brain can be damaged. The damage can lead to a loss of smell. Anosmia can be temporary or permanent. Medical researchers have been studying possible links between chemicals that gain access to the olfactory system, such as by inhalation of vapors or dusts, and the loss of smell. The loss of the sense of smell can be life-threatening because if you lose your sense of smell you will not be able to detect dangerous chemicals—during a gas leak, for example.

The loss of your sense of smell could signal problems with your brain, including some neurodegenerative diseases.[3] "Researchers at the University of Pennsylvania School of Medicine have linked smell loss in mice with excessive levels of a key protein associated with Alzheimer's and Parkinson's disease. Smell loss is well documented as one of the early and first clinical signs of such diseases. If smell function declines as the levels of this protein increase in brain regions associated with smelling, the research could validate the use of smell tests for diagnosing Alzheimer's disease.

" 'The loss of smell—or olfactory dysfunction—has been known for more than a decade as an early sign of several neurodegenerative diseases, but we have never been able to link it to a pathological entity that is measurable over time,' said Richard Doty, PhD, Professor and Director of Penn's Smell and Taste Center, who is also the team leader of the study. 'By tying decrements in the ability to smell to the presence of key disease proteins, such as tau, we may well be able to assess the degree of progression of selected elements of Alzheimer's disease and related disorders by scores on quantitative smell tests.' "[4]

Another article added schizophrenia, multiple sclerosis, and systemic lupus erythematosus (SLE), "an autoimmune disease that sometimes involves the central nervous system in a condition known as neuropsychiatric SLE (NPSLE). Research in mice has shown that NPSLE-like symptoms and olfactory impairment might be induced by autoimmune mechanisms that target specific areas of the brain, but this has not been explored. A new study assessed olfactory function in SLE patients and found that there is a decrease in the sense of smell compared with healthy controls."[5]

Although everyone tends to slowly lose their sense of smell as they age, scratch and sniff tests have been developed for doctors to use to determine if someone is losing their sense of smell earlier than normal.[6]

There is a zone on your face called the danger triangle.[7] It extends from the two corners of your mouth up to the top of your nose and includes your nose. Infections that develop in this area can, though rarely, flow directly to your brain via the blood supply and the cavernous sinus. Even infections of your upper front teeth are included in this danger triangle.

To protect yourself from infections in your nose, remember to never rinse your nasal passageways with water that has not been prescribed for that purpose. There is an ameba that is commonly found in soil and warmer waters called *Naegleria fowleri* that can gain access to your brain through your nose. This ameba, once in the brain, can lead to primary amebic meningoencephalitis, which destroys brain tissue, and causes death. People can be exposed while swimming.

What can you do? First, make sure that any water that enters your nose is safe, such as sterile saline water designed and sold for that purpose. Second, protect against infections in the danger triangle on your face. See a doctor early on if you have questions about possible infected sites. And, as mom always said, don't pick your nose.

On a more fun level, you can keep track of your ability to smell as you get older. Select foods that have distinct smells,

107

such as canned corn, sliced apples, peaches, and peeled bananas. Avoid foods with spicy type sensations, such as onion and clove, as these can trick you into thinking you smell them when it is not their smell that you are detecting. Outdoor items such as roses and cut grass have a strong and distinctive odor. Keep a diary of your smell observations every year. Make notes as to how strongly these things smell to you: strong smelling, easy to smell, difficult to smell, can't smell. If you notice a trend of loss in smell function, talk to your doctor about it.

Meanwhile, keep your nose clean, but let's not keep the importance of nose health a secret!

| 20 |

Know How Your Meds Affect Your Brain

Medicines can be your best friend or worst foe.

—Unknown

There is no doubt that medication can be a great ally in our quest to live a high-quality life. Medicines have usually been associated with cure or symptom relief and taken with little thought about adverse effects. But the truth is that as more and more exotic drugs are discovered every year and made available in prescription form or over the counter, some are having unwelcome and even dangerous side effects. Add to that the growing search for herbals to enhance our quest for good health and we have a potential lurking menace. Most of us can avoid a dangerous outcome just by discussing all the medicines and herbals we are consuming with our health care provider who can then, with his/her expertise and advanced medication software, help us guard against bad outcomes. Pharmacists are also taking up the challenge by putting time and energy into providing educational materials designed to alert us to potential problems with any new medicine. However, as gerontologists search for ways to avoid the traps of aging, they are becoming concerned about the fact that 50 percent of the adult population use medicines every day that could have negative effects on their aging brains.

Laura was determined to do all she could to stay sharp mentally and had heard so many testimonials about herbal medicines that she decided to try one of the popular ones. Unfortunately she did not check with her doctor, and she took an herbal with blood thinning properties along with her daily Coumadin. She soon developed slight oozing into her brain that required a hospital admission to control. Laura recovered but now, much wiser, only takes herbal medicines with her physician's knowledge. We all need to follow her lead.

A very well-designed study at the University of Illinois determined that commonly used medications may produce cognitive impairment in older adults. Some medications routinely used to treat medical conditions associated with aging (such as allergies, hypertension, asthma, and cardiovascular disease) appear to affect the brain in negative ways. The drugs studied included very popular over-the-counter medicines like antihistamines, some antidepressants, sleep aids, itching remedies, and digestive and urinary tract aids.[1]

Sam developed severe allergies upon moving to a lush area of the country where beautiful trees and flowers flourished but caused him increasingly disturbing symptoms. He suffered from stuffy nose, headaches, and sinus pressure and turned to his local drugstore for relief. He was elated when the over-the-counter medicine did in fact give him relief from his symptoms. It wasn't long, however, before Sam began noticing he was having problems concentrating at work and his keen memory for names seemed to be diminishing. Concerned about his job performance, he went to his physician and learned that his "allergy medicine" was the culprit. A change to a different remedy restored his memory and concentration, and a grateful Sam learned to be cautious about treating symptoms on his own.

Rita was having financial difficulty after a fire had destroyed much of her family's home. The stress caused her to lose sleep every night. Although Rita was able to feel peace and calm after prayer and reading well-loved Scriptures, she would wake suddenly at 3 a.m. almost every night as her fears took on giant proportions in the quiet of her room. Friends and family were concerned as she looked more and more exhausted, and they convinced her to "go to the drugstore and get something for sleep!" Although she was not one to take medicines, she agreed and began taking one of the popular sleep medicines. It worked wonderfully until she began noticing memory problems. Rita feared the worst, convinced she had a brain tumor or Alzheimer's, but she summoned her courage and went to her physician for a checkup. After a battery of tests, Rita learned that her symptoms were caused by her over-the-counter self-prescribed medication. Rita's doctor explained, "Seniors have several bodily changes that can make some drugs like these even more risky. Aging often causes muscle mass to be replaced by body fat, and people over sixty-five are often slightly dehydrated due to diminished thirst signals. Also, seniors produce less acetylcholine, making the effects of these medicines greater." In 1991 a concerned Dr. Mark Beers and his U.S. team of twelve health experts compiled a list to determine which drugs should be used or avoided in ambulatory and nursing homes. They were concerned that seniors especially are at risk for developing negative outcomes which include falls, depression, or in some cases even death. The list was updated in 2003 and had the hoped-for result of reducing adverse drug reactions in elderly populations.[2]

I (Jim) am often concerned about elderly patients who are taking prescription medications for anxiety long-term, because the medication can sometimes build up in the body, making it necessary to adjust the dose downward to continue a safe range. Some common side effects in addition to memory and concentration problems are dry mouth, confusion, blurry vision, constipation, dizziness, and changes in bladder control. Driving can be negatively affected. Many herbals are a great benefit, but you must be certain they are not reacting with another medicine or herbal you may be taking. Patients with chronic pain often benefit from treatment in a pain clinic so that medication can be safely prescribed and monitored. "Addictive substances can activate the dopamine reward system, providing pleasure. . . . Chronic exposure to drugs leads to the suppression of reward circuits, increasing the amounts needed to get the same effect. The opiate system is involved in pain and anxiety relief. The cholinergic circuits—where nicotine acts—are involved in memory and learning. Cocaine acts at the noradrenergic receptors, which are involved in stress responses and anxiety."[3] Self-medicating with any of these potent drugs is like playing Russian roulette with your brain.

Recently *The Seattle Times* reported that "more die from drugs than traffic accidents. Drug overdoses now outpace traffic accidents as the leading cause of injury-related death in 16 states, including Washington, as use of prescription painkillers continues to rise."[4] In addition, the recent concern over the under-treatment of debilitating effects of chronic pain has ushered in an increase in the use of opioids, such as

OxyContin. According to the University of Washington, these opioids (OxyContin, Vicodin, and Percocet) are prescribed to one in five adults and one in ten adolescents annually. A study conducted by Group Health Cooperative concluded that the number of people taking opiates daily has risen from 2 to 4 percent. This translates to mean that one in twenty-five adults are now taking this class of drugs every day.[5] Patients taking opioids are carefully cautioned about the potential dangers of the medications' effect on driving and are advised to avoid the potentially deadly combination of pain medication and alcohol.

Treat medications with great respect and don't ever fall into the trap of manipulating your medications and dosages. Marilyn Monroe, Judy Garland, Alan Ladd, Dave Waymer, Heath Ledger, Anna Nicole Smith, and of course Michael Jackson, all stars whose careers ended in tragedy, will forever be a reminder of the potential deadly dangers of drugs.

| 21 |

Learn a New Language

A different language is a different vision of life.
—Federico Fellini, Italian film director

Many of us as children enjoyed watching a spy movie where the hero or heroine easily passes through enemy checkpoints by fluently speaking a foreign language. You may even have fantasized about being a bilingual world traveler. Now you think that time has slipped away from you and, with it, so has your fantasy. But not so fast! It turns out that learning another language might not only fulfill your childhood dream, it may provide your brain with a workout regimen that will help keep it sharp into the endgame of life. Learning a language exercises a unique part of the brain, and it is different for reading and for conversation. Like cross-training, it exercises a different set of "brain muscles."

People often dread studying a new language out of a fear of failure. But consider this; your fear of learning another language may be a learned response. Many a youngster has heard an adult, or even a parent, say that they would love to learn a new language but it was just too hard. And so, you think, "If it was too hard for mom and dad when they were my age, it's probably also too hard for me." What may have been true for them is not necessarily true for you. One of the largest and most reliable longitudinal health studies, conducted by the Boston University School of Medicine, was launched in 1948 and studied 5,209 healthy adults living in Framingham, Massachusetts. The original study, called "The Framingham Study," gave birth to a study of the children of those in the original study. Since 1971, this second study, which is called "The Framingham Offspring Study," has shown, among other things, that the "Framingham offspring perform approximately 1 standard deviation better than their parents on most memory tests administered at comparable ages, despite (on average) sharing the same genes."[1] In separate studies, it has been observed that the average IQ in the U.S. increases by about 3 points every decade.[2] The good news is that your parents' boundaries are not yours. You are likely to live longer[3] and, based on choices you can make, you can do it with a cognitively younger brain.

While it is true that young brains easily make new connections, which facilitates learning, a Johns Hopkins University team recently published a study demonstrating that new adult-born neurons have a youthful level of plasticity, but only for a limited time window. They observe that this "represent[s] not merely a replacement mechanism for lost neurons but instead an ongoing developmental process that continuously rejuvenates the mature nervous system by offering expanded capacity of plasticity in response to experience throughout life."[4]

115

Another barrier to learning a new language is that, as you have aged, you have unconsciously developed acute listening "filters" to help your brain focus in on those parts of verbal expressions that carry most of the meaning. The trick about learning a new language is accepting that the English "filters" that you have been training for decades may not serve you well when learning a new language, because the information is *carried differently*. So, be patient with yourself. It will take time to un-train your English filters and train your subconscious for new language filters.

Bobbie recalls, "Our language filters, as well as those of our patients, were certainly in place on our first day of clinic in American Samoa as we strove to cross the wide language barrier. Samoans are remarkable, gentle, and resilient people who were warm and receiving but many spoke little, if any, English. We, on the other hand, spoke no Samoan other than *talafa lava* (hello) and *tofa soifua* (goodbye)! That first day we quickly learned that if we were to make any progress toward helping our patients, we most definitely needed an interpreter to discern where the 'pain in the belly' was coming from. By the end of the week we had made many new friends and learned some pronunciations and meanings for this beautiful language. The children taught us some Samoan songs and we saw firsthand how much it means to a person of another culture when a visitor attempts to speak their native language. On our last day we were immersed in a Samoan church service where all attendees from youngest baby to eldest Auntie were dressed in white and we were blessed by hearing our familiar hymns and choruses sung in Samoan by the villagers."

Once you decide to learn a new language, you have some choices to make, which you can combine with other strategies for brain health, some of which are covered separately in this book. For example, social interaction is good for brain health. If you learn your language by going to evening school, perhaps at the local high school, you will be interacting with others who are also struggling to "unlearn" their English filters, just like you. It is okay to struggle. Make your new motto "No strain, no brain!" You and your fellow struggling students may form a new social network. So, commit yourself to fulfilling a childhood dream. Be an inspiration to your children and grandchildren. Best of all, it will be good for your brain, so break out those cross-training flash cards. Capice?

| 22 |

Learn to Paint

Only when he no longer knows what he is doing does the painter do good things.

—Edgar Degas

It seems obvious that artistic painting is not like doing math or working at puzzles. One reason that painting is so different is that it is grounded in a different region of the brain. There is a distinction between our "left brain" and our "right brain," in reference to the left and right hemispheres of the cerebral cortex. The left and right hemispheres each have their own manner of perceiving information and processing it. The right brain tends to provide intuition, spatial perception, and the capability to multitask. The left brain tends to provide language, logic, and cognition of details. But the left brain-right brain dichotomy is by no means ironclad, and varies from one individual to another. For example, while the left brain is referred to as the "language center" of the brain, this is only true for 93 percent of us.[1] And, for many tasks that people accomplish every day, the left and right side of the brain must cooperate efficiently to arrive at a correct answer or to decide on a proper course of action.[2] The effects of separating the right and left brain have been studied for years in what are known as "split brain" studies, for which Dr. Roger Sperry was awarded a Nobel Prize in 1981. As a corrective to particular forms of epilepsy, the neural bridge between the left and right hemispheres, the corpus callosum, was surgically cut. This is effective, because specific types of epilepsy are caused by frenetic inter-hemispheric miscommunication, much like a short circuit. In the 1960s, the surgical procedure was to disrupt the entire corpus callosum, creating a "split brain." Through studies of patients having that procedure, science gained some definitive insights into the distinctions of left and right brain function in a large and otherwise healthy population. Today, modern medical methods allow the spot of the communication short circuit (i.e. the cause of the epilepsy) to be pinpointed and only that section of the neural bridge is surgically disrupted.

Many of the chapters in this book deal with brain functions rooted in left brain activities (e.g., cognition, logic, reasoning, and language). The strategies presented in this book for improving or preserving brain health are supported by referenced and peer-reviewed scientific articles. Most of these strategies target left brain health and performance. Studies on right brain health are more difficult to find. This may be because the functions of the right brain are harder to measure (e.g., how well does someone perceive spatial orientation, use imagination, or intuit emotions), and science is grounded in measuring things. It is also true that medical science must follow the demand signal of grant funding. The reality is that our Western culture is much more interested in left brain health and performance than in that of the right brain. In other words, math and engineering are valued over art and music. Education reform is centered on the "3Rs" (reading, writing, and arithmetic, which are largely left brain activities) and art is relegated to the proverbial back seat.

An incisive, thought-provoking article, published in early 2010, helps us understand this "swing of the pendulum":

> With the Reformation, and with the beginnings of the Enlightenment, there [was] a shift in mentality towards what is certain, rigid, fixed and simplified. Ambiguity was no longer a sign of richness, but of obscurity. Imagination was mistrusted and metaphor became a lie. As Descartes said, things can be seen clearly only if they are seen singly, one by one. The world was atomized. And with these developments came a rise in the mechanical model as the only framework for understanding ourselves and the world.
>
> This led to our own age, to a world where the right hemisphere, with its broader view, has been systematically discounted. Like the brain itself, the battle I describe is asymmetrical. Each swing of the pendulum has carried us further into the territory of the left hemisphere's world.
>
> The two hemispheres also differ in their attitude to their differences. The right hemisphere is inclusive in its attitude to what the left hemisphere might know, but the left hemisphere is exclusive of the right. Where the right hemisphere's world responds to negative feedback, the left hemisphere gets locked ever further into its own point of view.
>
> And so our world has become increasingly rule-bound. Loss of the implicit damages our ability to convey, or even to see at all, aspects of ourselves and our world that transcend the mechanistic. Perspective in art has receded along with harmony in music: We tend more and more to see the world as a heap of intrinsically meaningless fragments.[3]

Lance is a pastor. He is a bit "tightly strung" and he knows this. Lance decided to take up painting as a form of therapy. He had always wanted to learn to paint, so he thought, *Why not give it a try?* To avoid the stress of taking classes, he decided to take up paint-by-number painting. He had a lot of stress, so he did a lot of painting. After the walls in his house were covered with his artwork, the completed canvasses began to fill up his attic. Along the way, he developed some painting skills. He developed comfort with the brush. He learned how perspective was created on the canvas. He learned use of color. He learned what it was about a painting that pleased him. One day, Lance realized that he had changed. He wanted to choose his own subject matter and began painting on blank canvases. His works are now more than therapeutic; they are expressions of his inner self. His paintings give him pleasure and his occasional art shows are crowd pleasers.

For Lance, painting started as left brain activity of following instructions and working within defined boundaries, moving sequentially from one pre-drawn shape to another. Eventually, he integrated a strong right brain collaboration that was free of boundaries and instructions. His right brain imagined the whole, even while his left brain focused on the individual parts. Lance became an artist, painting what he wanted and how he wanted and doing it very well.

Right brain health is more than just the ability to appreciate or create art. Intuition tells you that a healthy right brain is important to a good life. In a study of patients with injured frontal lobes (part of the cerebral cortex), the patients with left lobe injuries were compared to patients having right lobe injuries. A test was administered, known as a rule-switching test. A rule-switching test is designed to cause people to make mistakes. Those with left frontal lobe injuries corrected 68 percent of their errors, while those with right lobe injuries corrected only 30 percent.[4] How the left and right brain perceive and interpret information is very different, and what the right brain contributes can be very important to everyday life.

Jill Bolte Taylor is a neuroanatomist, who at the age of thirty-seven suffered a stroke that traumatized the left side of her brain. She lost the ability to walk, talk, read, write, or recall any portion of her life. After successful surgery to remove a clot and several years of rehab, Jill enjoyed a full recovery. She wrote about her experience in *My Stroke of Insight: A Brain Scientist's Personal Journey*. In it, she extols to virtues of embracing right brain perceptions and processing. On the lecture circuit, she challenges her audiences to pursue right brain thinking as the key to happy living.

Each of us is free (to some degree) to choose whether we favor our left or our right brain in dealing with daily life. Most of us do not even consider this a choice. We have developed a pattern of living that thoughtlessly favors one side over the other. Our post-industrial culture rewards left brain thinking, and for the most part, we are products of our culture. But consider the old expression "remember to stop and smell the roses." This is a call to make choices that are outside of our default patterns of living. While the originator of this expression probably did not know it, smelling the roses would first require the right brain to identify the rose; the left brain would be trying to ruin the moment by cataloging the number of petals, the height of the pistil, the length of the sepals, and so forth.

Students of art are often fascinated by the journey artists take as they explore and express various techniques through their paintings. Artists' creations are windows into their mind and soul and often tell their own unique life story. In this sense, a picture really can be worth a thousand words, for as the famous preacher Henry Ward Beecher said, "Every artist dips his brush in his own soul, and paints his own nature into his pictures."[5]

If your life is full of details, sequential tasks, financial analysis, and learning, you may be living a left-brain dominant life. Living life to the fullest may require thoughtful choices to unleash the unique power of right brain perception and processing. Maybe it is time for you to stop and smell the roses. When you are done smelling them, it may be time for you to pull up an easel and paint them as well.

| 23 |

Memorize

Memory moderates prosperity, decreases adversity, controls youth, and delights old age.

—Anonymous[1]

Memory researchers prove again and again that our brains are far from stagnant. They can change, grow, and repair themselves at surprising rates of speed. Memory is important to us not only because it catalogues our life events but also because being able to remember enhances our ability to think on higher levels. It is good news to know that losing our memory is not necessarily a *result* of aging but can *accompany* it. Therefore it is wise and worthwhile to devote some time and energy to memorizing and keeping our brain sharp.

I (Bobbie) am laughing as I write this chapter because we just moved to yet another new apartment and we are struggling to memorize which drawer holds the silverware, which way to turn to find the bathroom in the middle of the night, and the location of all the light switches. Sounds easy, right? Trust us, it isn't! At least not when you have to do it multiple times every year.

Our phenomenal brains are not only capable of memorizing new surroundings, but of reconstructing past experiences. Whether you are attempting to learn to ride a bike, remember the beloved face of your great grandmother, or find the silverware drawer, all of these challenges have two things that are necessary for success: learning and reconstructing the past. Learning is a process whereby a group of neurons fire at the same time, producing an experience. The neuronal pathway is changed so that in the future these same neurons are more likely to fire together. Repeating this cycle makes it easier to "recall" and reproduce the skill being learned.

Memories are made as we flow through three steps. First of course we must pay attention long enough to learn new information, which is then stored into temporary nerve-cell pathways. Most researchers believe that the first few seconds of storing a new memory take place in the sensory part of our brains. Our amazing brains automatically record touch, scent, taste, sound, or visual cues of the moment; then the new memory is placed into short-term storage. Memories are actually stored in bits and pieces distributed throughout the brain. Each memory is made up of a web of sensory information and fact. Our memory "software" is created in such a way that it makes long-term memories less destructible. For instance, the memory of a beloved dog may be sparked when we see an animal of the same breed, and unique aspects of our pet will often come flooding back, such as the silkiness of his reddish-brown coat, the sparkle in his brown eyes, and his excited yelp as he headed to the front door for a walk. Researchers have found that the hippocampus in the brain triggers this memory web of neurons that are emotionally charged or well-learned and retrieves the short- or long-term memory.[2]

The hippocampus is also believed to be in charge of determining if a memory should be saved. This tiny seahorse-shaped "judge" will screen out those occurrences that seem immaterial. Is it important to remember how many trees were swaying in the wind outside your window? Probably not. But what about how much computer paper is left? Yes, this should be retained at least long enough to make it to your shopping list. If a memory pathway is not strengthened it will quickly fade; it must be reinforced in order to eventually find its way into long-term storage where it will have staying power. If the memory is associated with a strong emotion like fear, or better yet, joy, it will be easier to retain. This is in part due to the body chemicals that are secreted during emotional times. High levels of stress or sleep deprivation, on the other hand, greatly impede our ability to remember.

The third phase of memory function is the retrieval phase. When we recall the memory, it comes back by way of the nerve pathways, and the more frequently we recall it, the better it is remembered. Most of us remember learning our multiplication tables, which have years of staying power, and most would agree the process was tinged with at least a low dose of stress!

Researchers have found that when we do take the time to memorize new things it promotes neuron growth and actually creates new brain connections. The myelin sheaths that cover and protect our neural pathways are strengthened and the brain itself actually grows in size, giving us extra thinking capacity.[3] The hippocampus is not only important in memory recall but also is crucial in navigation. When we move around, neurons (known as place cells) activate to tell us where we are. This process is known as spatial memory.[4]

I (Jim) certainly hope to keep this part of my brain healthy as we sprint across the country several times a year to various medical assignments. I learned early on to focus attention on the necessities during those first few weeks in a new setting. Anyone who has made a major move can appreciate the number of new habits and changes that need to be jump-started. For instance, I remember feeling a bit overwhelmed as we drove out of the Denver airport in our unfamiliar rental car into six busy, blaring lanes of traffic. I was thinking how much I would miss my previous leisurely drive to work along country roads! Over the next few days I had to learn not only the location of the windshield wipers but also the location of my new hospital, apartment, grocery store, pharmacy, parking spot, as well as computer passwords and software, while making sense of the maze of corridors in the new hospital. It would be *mind-boggling* if I had not learned a few memory survival tricks along the way:

- Forget what you no longer need to remember to make room for new "survival items."
- Clear away distractions and really *focus* on the new information.
- Make associations to jog your memory (i.e. attach a visual image to new names or directions).
- Designate a place to keep your "gear" (cell phone, keys, and in my case beeper and stethoscope).
- Be willing to re-learn each day until the new info is entrenched in your memory bank.
- Don't get discouraged; instead, celebrate that you are giving your brain a great workout.

Memory is a fascinating topic and much is being learned as researchers continually study its many facets. For instance, state-dependant memory shows the versatility of how memories are made. This type of memory is laid down when we are in a specific situation. For instance, it has been discovered that students who study for exams while drinking are unable to recall the information as readily or correctly when sober. They are only able to recall some of the facts they studied while inebriated. On a more positive note, our friend Janice experienced the richness of state-dependant memory through an unexpected experience. She had been brought up in the church but after graduation got involved in a busy life that did not include church attendance. Then, many years later, she happened to be walking past a church one snowy evening and, hearing Christmas carols, was drawn inside. Immediately the candlelight, scent of fresh cut pine, and view of the choir dressed in their robes brought back a flood of wonderful childhood memories. She found a "new church home" that night along with a host of new friends.

Remember. The brain is constantly changing and enriching our lives and can be tuned up with use. Many seventy-year-olds perform as well on certain cognitive tests as twenty-year-olds, and verbal intelligence tends to improve as we age. So get started and memorize a new quote or song today. Here's one to start: "Consult not your fears but your hopes and your dreams. Think not about your frustrations, but about your unfulfilled potential. Concern yourself not with what you tried and failed in, but with what it is still possible for you to do" (Pope John XXIII).

| 24 |

Mind Your Head

Traumatic brain injury (TBI) is the leading cause of death and disability in Americans under the age of 45.[1]

The first time I (Dave) saw the ubiquitous UK warning sign, "Mind Your Head," it took me awhile to figure out I should duck. Maybe a sign with a duck on it might have worked better in my case.

On September 26, 2009, millions of U.S. college football fans held their collective breath when the seemingly invincible Tim Tebow, senior quarterback for the Florida "Gators," took a hit in the backfield that left him on his back, unconscious, with a concussion serious enough to cause vomiting and observation in a hospital. Thankfully, Tebow, the homeschooled son of former missionaries, seemed to recover quickly enough to play again two weeks later, and then took his team to an undefeated regular season before losing in the SEC Championship game to Alabama.

Concussions occur when the brain is slammed into the inside of the skull, disrupting normal brain activity. They occur with regularity in football, despite recent advances in equipment and changes in the rules. NeurosurgeryToday.org estimates that among high school, college, and professional players the number of concussions is 300,000 annually.[2] Until relatively recently, this effect was more or less shrugged off as a part of a hard-hitting game that only "real men" should play until they couldn't take it anymore.

One of the formerly overlooked long-term effects of concussions, especially multiple concussions, is depression. For example, retired Super Bowl champion linebacker Ted Johnson experienced at least fifty concussions during his career, always returning to the game as quickly as possible. He retired, in part due to his depression, which was severe enough to keep him in bed, in the dark, for the better part of a year and a half.[3]

Dementia is another, much worse, possible long-term result of concussion. John Mackey, a football star receiver with the Baltimore Colts under Johnny Unitas, scored a seventy-five-yard touchdown in 1971 to help the Colts win Super Bowl V. Later, he was inducted into the Pro Football Hall of Fame. But today, the fame means little to either Mackey or his wife, who had to appeal to the NFL for help with the high cost of caring for John's severe dementia, symptoms of which began to exhibit themselves when Mackey, now sixty-eight, was in his early fifties. Mackey is one of about a hundred former players with severe dementia receiving help from what is called the "88 plan," in honor of John's jersey number. The fund provides up to $88,000 annually toward the cost of their care.

Interviewed on the CBS show *60 Minutes*, Dr. Robert Cantu (originator of the Cantu Concussion Guidelines, which is the current test used to evaluate the severity of sports concussions) believes it will eventually be proven that the problems of Mackey and many of these players were caused by the hits they took on the field. "In reality, I suspect if their brains could be studied, and hopefully one day they will, that traumatic encephalopathy is what has caused this dementia," he said. The NFL has recently mandated that an independent neurologist would determine when a player with a head injury can return to the game.[4]

Yet 300,000 football-related concussions are just the tip of the iceberg of such injuries from all sports and recreation activities combined. There are between five and twelve times that number (1.6 to 3.8 million) of sports and recreation-related concussions annually in the United States, according to the CDC's National Center for Injury Prevention and Control.[5] In addition to football, these would include organized sports like soccer, baseball and softball, boxing, competitive cycling, hockey, horseback riding, racing motor vehicles, skiing, wrestling, martial arts, and pole vaulting. Some of these require protective headgear, some do not. Yet sometimes even protective headgear does not protect the way one might expect.

Purely recreational forms of some of the above sports can result in brain trauma, with or without a helmet. Plus there are many other recreational activities that can produce a closed head brain injury, including bicycle riding, kayaking, skateboarding, snow skiing, snowboarding, surfboarding, sailboarding, rock climbing, rollerblading, and water skiing—any recreational activity in which your head can receive a hard enough knock or jolt for your brain to collide with the inside of your skull. You don't even have to actually hit your head on anything. What matters is what happens between the outside of your brain and the inside of your skull. This was tragically illustrated by the death of actress Natasha Richardson, who died in March 2009 as a result of a fall while learning to ski in Montreal. She was not wearing a helmet, but reports stated that she did not actually strike her head on anything, or show any sign of external injury.

I (Dave) can attest to the possibility of brain injury without impact, having experienced this in the fall of 2008 when I fell backward while loading a trailer. I didn't actually strike my head on the floor; but I did become very ill with the typical symptoms of concussion, including severe vomiting and even diarrhea concurrently. I thought I had eaten some tainted food. But Ms. Richardson's death and subsequent reflection and study into closed head injuries helped me realize what had really happened—and how fortunate I had been not to have left this life before we could finish this book.

Despite the high incidence of head injuries from recreation and organized sports, the top three leading causes of head injuries in America are: auto accidents (passengers or pedestrians); bicycle and motorcycle accidents; and falls (children and especially the elderly).[6]

- More than 50 percent of head injuries yearly are associated with automobiles. Approximately 50,000 children are hit by cars. Most passenger injuries are due to lack of proper use of seat belts and child safety restraints.

- Only 20 percent of children in the U.S. wear helmets while bike riding. Of the 350,000 children involved in bike-related accidents annually, 130,000 sustain head injuries.

- In states without helmet laws, only 20 to 25 percent of bikers and 28 to 40 percent of motorcyclists wear helmets. Motorcyclists are fourteen times more likely to die in a crash and three times more likely to incur a head injury. This in spite of the fact that The National Highway Traffic Safety Administration (NHTSA) says helmets are 85 to 88 percent effective in preventing head injuries.

- Falls are also among the top ten injuries that bring young children to ERs. The most frequent falls are in playgrounds, from walkers, shopping carts, and windows (kids can fall through a five-inch opening in windows).
- Falls are the leading cause of head injuries for the elderly. In fall-related deaths, 60 percent are seventy-five or older. Many seniors have problems with balance and environmental hazards such as uneven floors, loose rugs, unstable furniture, and poor lighting. In 2003, 1.8 million seniors sixty-five and over were treated in the ER for falls; over 421,000 were hospitalized.[7]

Another significant but underreported cause of brain injury is due to combat. According to the Brain Trauma Foundation, blasts are a leading cause of TBI among active duty military personnel in war zones. Veterans' advocates believe that between 10 and 20 percent of Iraq veterans, or between 150,000 and 300,000 service members, have some level of TBI. Thirty percent of soldiers admitted to Walter Reed Army Medical Center have suffered traumatic brain injuries.[8]

The long-term impact of head injuries is significant:

- At least 5.3 million Americans, 2 percent of the U.S. population, currently live with disabilities resulting from TBI.
- Moderate and severe head injury (respectively) are associated with a 2.3 and 4.5 times increased risk of Alzheimer's disease.
- Direct medical costs and indirect costs such as lost productivity of TBI totaled an estimated $60 billion in the

United States in 2000.[9] Surely in 2010 that cost will be substantially higher.

Sometimes the long-term effect of a closed head traumatic brain injury can be catastrophic for the person injured and his or her family and wider circle of friends:

Jenny Grogan was the kind of kid you would want your son to marry. Outgoing, attractive, athletic, intelligent, funny— she loved to laugh and she loved to live. When her parents sent her off to college, they were confident she would find success in whatever field she decided to pursue. Then something happened. Midway through her freshman year, Jenny was playing goalie in an indoor soccer game, and in her "full-throttle" mode she dove to block a kick, only to hit her head very hard, too hard, on the hardwood gym floor. She caught her breath, and then continued to play. Later that night, she began to feel nauseous, a little dizzy, with a significant headache. So she visited the campus infirmary, where the doctor gave her a cursory exam, and sent her back to the dorm with some medication for the pain. Within a few months, Jenny's disposition had changed from mostly sunny to cloudy with thunderstorms, daily. Her grades dropped, her new friends wondered what was happening, and she gradually developed the symptoms of depression, leaving school midterm to return home where she hoped to sort it out. She never did. Baffling everyone who had ever known her, including her parents, in the end, Jenny took her own life.

So, whatever your age (or your kids' ages) make sure you protect your brain from jolts and knocks. Wear that helmet, even if it seems uncool. Click that seat belt, even if you think you'll never need it. And always remember that your brain is far more sensitive to trauma than you can possibly imagine.

| 25 |

Pay Attention to the Brain in Your Gut

You have to master not only the art of listening to your head, you must also master listening to your heart and to your gut.

—Carly Fiorina[1]

Surprise! Your gut has a brain of its own that powers up and controls many of your digestive functions. This amazing system is called the "Enteric Nervous System" (ENS) and is located all through the lining of the GI tract. It communicates with the brain via the spinal cord. The ENS "talks to" the brain in our head by way of a small number of command neurons, which allow it to both send and receive messages. In fact, there is a lively conversation going on most of the day as situations and experiences open up a chat line between our two brains.

The ENS is made up of a network of neurons, proteins, and chemicals which allow it not only to learn and remember but also to produce our "gut feelings."[2] Have you ever had a "gut-wrenching" experience? Has an exchange of words with your boss made you feel nauseous? Have you pondered where the "butterflies" came from, or why people sometimes feel "choked with emotion"? Well here are some answers.

For the last twenty years or so gastroenterologists have been hard at work studying the intricate connections between the brain and the gut. The discoveries have amazed and convinced even the most skeptical and given birth to a fascinating new medical specialty called neuro-gastroenterology. One of the pioneers in this specialty, Dr. Douglas Drossman from the University of North Carolina, is considered the world authority in his field and has written over 400 books, articles, and abstracts. His research and treatment discoveries have given hope to countless patients suffering from disturbing stress-related brain-gut symptoms. A recent publication on the *patient's* perspective highlights the critical importance of good communication and understanding between patients and the doctor as well as relatives and friends. The study confirms again the important role that decreasing stress and promoting good relationships plays in improving quality of life.[3]

As a gastroenterologist, I (Jim) want to give you an insider's look at how these complex brain-gut interactions occur. The gut contains 100 million neurons and is connected to the brain by layers of specialized tissue. The vagus nerve is the stick shift and controls the volume of gastrointestinal activity. The gut is not only able to *send* signals to the brain but *receives* information and "requests" as well. It also acts as a sort of drug store for the body's needs. The enteric nervous system can dispense major neurotransmitters like dopamine and serotonin as well as various endorphins (the body's natural tranquilizers) at a moment's notice. Also located throughout the GI tract are brain proteins, sensors, neuron nourishers, and immune system cells needed for various body functions. With every meal we eat, the enteric nervous system springs into action to monitor the digestion process and determine how your chicken and mashed potatoes should be mixed and propelled. This is often the reason we are highly tuned in to our gut messages when negative information like pain and bloating make their way to our brain.

Our modern way of life is often filled with stressful situations. In fact, 20 percent of our U.S. population suffers from a stress-related brain-gut condition called Irritable Bowel Syndrome (IBS). Stress signals from the brain can alter nerve function and turn up the volume of serotonin circuits in the gut. This over-stimulation can cause problems all through the GI tract such as trouble swallowing, heartburn, nausea, abdominal pain, altered bowel habits, or bloating. Thankfully, these symptoms can be successfully treated now that physicians better understand the causes. In bygone days when patients were told, "All your tests are normal," they sometimes feared they were just imagining these debilitating symptoms or worse yet the doctor had somehow missed a cancer that was still lurking. Unfortunately this can lead to depression in some cases as sufferers feel helpless when there seems to be no good treatment plan to calm down their GI tract and help them lead a more normal life.

Dr. Drossman and others, armed with the valuable new research knowledge, have dedicated much of their time and energy to devising lifestyle changes that in many cases allow patients to live symptom-free the majority of the time. Once patients with severe symptoms have been tested to be sure there are no signs of cancer or inflammatory bowel disease the doctor can confidently attribute the symptoms to IBS.

Here are a few of the recommendations that often bring relief to those diagnosed with Irritable Bowel Syndrome:

1. Stop smoking as it causes stimulation of the GI tract.
2. Drink only small amounts of alcohol if you drink at all as this irritates the GI tract.
3. Avoid saturated fat, roughage, dairy products, and caffeine for 2 to 3 weeks and see if it helps your symptoms. Take Metamucil every day while on this regimen. Slowly add back into your diet those foods you eliminated to see which seem to trigger symptoms for you.
4. Drink plenty of water.
5. Learn stress reduction techniques and don't hesitate to get counseling to help with difficult problems.
6. Exercise regularly as this reduces stress hormones and encourages healthy digestion and elimination.
7. Join a healthy church community and surround yourself with positive people who pray for you.
8. Log on to www.helpforibs.org for additional tips.

Jerry was a fifty-two-year-old worker for the United States Postal Service. He had been employed there for more than ten years, but a distressing set of physical symptoms was making it more and more difficult to perform his work. He had developed severe diarrhea along with abdominal cramping and was miserable at the prospect of having to stop numerous times while driving throughout the day to use a roadside restroom. Fearing he had cancer, Jerry finally agreed to see a physician. I (Jim) did a few tests and thankfully found no sign of tumors or inflammatory diseases. I sat down with Jerry and said, "Jerry you are free of disease but have a classic case of Irritable Bowel Syndrome. This chronic brain-gut condition is what is causing your symptoms. Have you been under more stress lately?"

"Well," admitted Jerry, "come to think about it, the symptoms started around the time the Post Office cut back on personnel and my work load skyrocketed. At the same time we also found my daughter needed surgery."

"It is not unusual that this extra stress was enough to trigger all your uncomfortable GI symptoms," I replied.

"Wow! I just am shocked to find out that there is a connection. I had no idea," he said.

"Let's get you started on medication and some dietary guidelines and see if we can get these symptoms quickly under control."

Jerry also agreed to see a counselor for some stress-reduction sessions. Within a month, Jerry's symptoms had started to improve and he was his happy-go-lucky self once again, no longer dreading each day of work.

Then there was Wes. He was a high-powered, successful young trial lawyer who came to see me when his pain and severe diarrhea were undermining his ability to function at his best in the courtroom. He had no idea what was causing his distressing symptoms, but he did know that without help his career would suffer. Testing revealed there was no structural damage or disease. suggesting that Wes, too, was suffering from IBS. He remembered that his dad had also experienced these symptoms, but back then there was no known way to alleviate the symptoms other than to take a strong medication that made him too sleepy to do his job. I was glad to be able to start Wes on a treatment plan and soon got a call from him reporting that he was free of symptoms and able to get back on track with his court cases.

The moral of these stories is: If your gut starts "complaining," scc your doctor and get some help to restore peaceful communication between the brain in your gut and the one inside your skull.

| 26 |

Play Mind-Friendly Games

Ninety-five percent of this game is half mental.

—Yogi Berra, baseball legend[1]

Of course we know that Yogi Berra was talking about baseball, but did you know that playing games—board games, word games, card games, crossword puzzles, and computer games—is also good for your cognitive functions? So if you want to increase your mental powers and help ward off dementia and Alzheimer's, consider dusting off your chessboard, checkerboard, dominos, or Scrabble game and going a few rounds with your family and friends.

Having a sharp mind and a strong memory depends on the "vitality of your brain's network of interconnecting neurons, and especially on junctions between these neurons called synapses. Since many of the brain changes that accompany aging and mental disorders are associated with deterioration or loss of synapses, learning ways to strengthen and protect these important connections may help you delay or avoid cognitive decline."[2]

Research has shown that a lack of stimulation is associated with a reduced number of synaptic connections in the brain. One study suggests that seniors who enjoy a variety of intellectually challenging activities, such as playing games and solving puzzles, have a lower risk of developing dementia.[3] The secret is to vary your mental activities and not let them become rote or routine. In other words, if you are a crossword puzzle whiz and can do them while you sleep, you might want to add something else to your repertoire, such as word or number games, to keep yourself mentally challenged and learning something new. Anything that relies on logic, word skills, math, and so on will help improve your brain's speed and memory. There are hundreds of online games, ranging from solitaire and other card games, to puzzles and word games, which can keep you mentally stimulated and challenged as you perfect your skills.

Bill and Mona both had challenging careers, so when they decided to move into a retirement community they wanted to stay sharp mentally as well as physically. Mona described their strategy. "In addition to playing tennis several times a week," she said, "Bill and I seized the opportunities all around us to stay challenged mentally. There are games and puzzles everywhere! As we wait for the elevator, we fit a few pieces into the 'puzzle in progress' located in each residence. There are Wii tournaments in our retirement residence, and we all try our hand at sports or even try learning to play an instrument. Opportunities for card and computer games abound. Recently something new has been started here at Shell Point Retirement Community (Ft. Myers, Florida) that has everyone talking. It is a five-week-long seminar on the brain! It is amazing how popular the class is. One friend went to the first class and said they could not wait 'til the second. It is so exciting and popular they hope to introduce it throughout the entire state. They will even train you to be a teacher!

"A book called *The Memory Bible*, by Gary Small, was recommended and Bill and I are going to the bookstore to get it this week. The teachers suggest that all of us should get a memory test, which is covered by Medicare. After all, we go for all kinds of physical tests, so why not include memory? I think it is a good idea, so I am going to encourage Bill to go and we can take it together. In addition to all this, our retirement community is going to introduce their plans for 'Big Brain Academy,' based on Nintendo software. One of our friends already started. He said his driving improved a great deal after doing the program regularly. He also was thrilled to find his focus and concentration improving. Another friend said their ability to do Sudoku improved. I am definitely going to volunteer to help out!"

How about video games? They're not just for kids anymore. Scientists are beginning to recognize the cognitive benefits of playing video games: pattern recognition, system thinking, and even patience. The theory is that gaming can exercise the mind the way physical activity exercises the body, and that it builds rather than diminishes cognitive skills.[4]

If you "Google" brain training and fitness websites, you will find several that have a variety of games and activities. Lumosity and Happy Neuron offer a variety of challenging games and activities for a small monthly fee. Many sites are free. Of course games can be addicting just as anything else can be, but the goal here is to challenge your brain, to improve short-term memory and concentration, and to have fun in the process.

Many "seniors" have discovered the benefit of solving riddles, doing word puzzles, and mental math—"brain jogging," that helps us to think critically and stay sharp. These activities can also be a good way to meet others and to work as a team. So have fun online, or look for a brain workshop near you!

| **27** |

Practice Positive Self-Talk

Every waking moment we talk to ourselves about the things we experience. Our self-talk, the thoughts we communicate to ourselves, in turn control the way we feel and act.

—John Lembo[1]

We all have days when we are down. Sometimes it's hard to maintain a positive outlook when our job is demanding, the kids are sick, the dishwasher breaks down after a big meal, there are bills to pay and very little money, and on and on. This happens to all of us. It's easy to have a glass-half-empty attitude when that's how the glass looks. In reality, however, this glass-half-empty outlook is not good for your health— physically, mentally, socially, or spiritually:

A positive outlook is one of the most important things we can do to keep our brains healthy and ready for learning. How we view ourselves, how we perceive the world around

144

us, and how we interact with others can have profound effects on our overall well-being and on our brains. . . .

Studies that chronicled lifestyle factors of people who stayed mentally sharp into old age showed that feeling good about ourselves and having a sense of self-worth and effectiveness in our lives are pillars of successful aging. Also important is maintaining a degree of control over our lives and to feel as if we are contributing to our families and society. Research shows that older adults may naturally tune into the positive aspects of life. A study at Stanford University, using a variation of the MRI to track patterns of activity in the brain, found that older adults are more responsive to positive images than to negative ones.[2]

Having a positive attitude, therefore, is important to you no matter what your current age or present situation. But, how do you manage this—on good days and bad days? How do you develop a glass-half-full outlook on life? It all goes back to your brain and reprogramming your thinking. Where do our negative and positive thoughts come from?

They are based on our beliefs and are formed early in life. They are influenced by the beliefs we have about ourselves and those that others have about us. Beliefs, then, influence our thoughts, which influence our self-talk, which ultimately influences our attitudes and behaviors.

We need to examine our inner messages and our beliefs—that is, what we think and believe about ourselves and the world around us. It is important to examine our feelings about particular thoughts and to decide if those thoughts are *true* or *untrue*. The more true and real a thought is and the better you feel about it, the more you can make those thoughts occur with greater frequency.

For example, Sharon grew up in a very abusive home. She was an unwanted child who was frequently told she was useless and would never amount to anything. She believed this throughout her childhood and into her adult life *even after* she got her master's degree in education and became a very successful drama teacher, raised three very well adjusted and successful sons, and had a happy marriage. It was difficult for Sharon to believe that she was successful and worthwhile because of the messages she heard as a child. Her self-talk and behavior was often degrading to herself. It was only after several years of therapy that she learned how to stop those negative thoughts and to replace them with positive ones about herself. She has become a much happier, more positive person who can celebrate her successes because she knows she has earned them.

Negative thinking and self-talk often takes the form of black and white thinking; disqualifying the positive and focusing on the negative; magnifying your mistakes; feeling you should, ought to, or must; labeling yourself a loser when you make a mistake; filtering everything that happens through a negative filter; assuming negative emotions reflect the way things really are; and personalizing every event as though you are the cause of it. These are also known as "cognitive distortions" or distorted thought patterns.

It is also important that you don't undermine positive thinking with such ideas as, "I never do anything right," or "I am so stupid." Replace these phrases with more positive ones. "Sometimes I do stupid things, but I'm basically a smart person."

What are the advantages of developing positive thought patterns, which lead to positive self-talk and positive behavior? "There is a science that is emerging that says positive self-talk isn't just a state of mind. It also has linkages to what's going on in the brain and in the body," said Carol Ryff, a psychology professor at the University of Wisconsin-Madison.[3]

Studies show that positive thinking and self-talk help you to sustain a healthy immune system, help bring more success in life, help you to live longer (studies show that optimists are 55 percent less likely to die from diseases than pessimists), help you to be healthier in general, help you to age more gracefully, protect your heart, and reduce stress.[4]

It's up to you. Take an active role in becoming more positive. Be proactive about things that happen and thoughts that pop into your mind. Don't just let life happen to you—take control of how you think about it, which determines how you feel about it, which then determines how you act. Look at yourself and life realistically, assess what's true and what's not, and then do what you have to do to change it.

And, finally, let your self-talk be guided by this Scripture: "There are some great things to think about, even though the world around us is so evil. Things that are true and good, lovely and honest, just and pure—these are the kind of thoughts that deserve your focus. Dwelling on these thoughts will produce mental and spiritual health and overall well-being in your life."[5]

| 28 |

Protect Your Brain from Insects

The smallest insect may cause death by its bite.

—Ancient Proverb[1]

When I (Dave) was about sixteen, I served as a counselor at a Christian camp not too far from my home in Vermont, where mosquitoes were more than just pests, though until then I never thought of them as mortal enemies. All counselors and campers were required to purchase a very inexpensive insurance policy, which most likely had to pay very few claims, since campers were there only a week at a time and our most risky contact sport was eating breakfast. But that year one camper had the misfortune of contracting "sleeping sickness" (equine encephalitis), which I had never heard about but have never forgotten since then. As it turned out, the pool and the stream that fed it were producing an impressive crop of mosquitoes that year, one of which had evidently dined upon a nearby horse that was infected with the eastern equine encephalomyelitis (EEE) virus, before it selected that particular camper for dessert. Equine encephalitis is preventable in horses, but not treatable in humans (about 35 percent of infected humans die from this illness). When the insurance company was forced to pay for that camper's care (I believe she developed a long-term disability), there was much ado about it in the camp, where we all engaged in a massive mosquito control effort, including closing and treating the pool and putting the brook off limits to all but the trout.

Since then (the mid-60s) several new insect-borne diseases with potential central nervous system (CNS) consequences have burst on the scene, including Lyme disease (tick-borne, discovered 1975) and the West Nile virus (mosquito-borne, discovered 1999). These, added to Rocky Mountain Spotted fever (tick-borne, discovered in the 1930s) now provide anyone informed in these matters just cause to either stay inside when the temperature is above freezing, or to ensure that they, and everyone they care about, are well protected when they venture forth into the insect empire known as the great outdoors. Several other insect-borne diseases with CNS consequences exist, but most of them are relatively rare in the U.S.

Lyme disease, named after the Connecticut town where it was first identified, is spread by ticks with an affinity for white-tail deer. According to the CDC, this disease affects about 16,000 people per year in the U.S., mostly in the northeastern, mid-Atlantic, and upper north-central regions, and in several counties in northwestern California.[2] Though it is treatable, especially early on, many cases are not recognized either by the patient or the healthcare provider until it is possible that there may be long-term CNS (and other) effects. Many people have been fighting this infection for years—some, like our teacher-friend Betsy, whose story follows, for more than thirty years, with significant ongoing health results.

Betsy writes:

I was resting, with my head down on my desk between classes, when a co-worker wandered in and announced, "You look awful!"

"Yeah, well, I'm not feeling too good," I replied.

"Again? Man, you're sick all the time!"

I decided that, as a teacher, I should take the high road and educate. "Lyme disease."

"Oh yeah, I forgot. But, how come you're still sick? You've been sick for years, haven't you?"

"Off and on, but the doctors think I had it for over thirty years before it was diagnosed. So it takes a while to knock it out."

I didn't want to admit that although Lyme disease can be cured, especially if caught right away, 20 percent of us continue to struggle for unknown reasons, with no end in sight. I wanted to defend myself by saying that I work a full-time job and a part-time job to pay my massive medical bills and for my meds, since the health insurance companies decided I was the equivalent of Typhoid Mary. I wanted to whine about having to sleep every second when it wasn't absolutely necessary to be dressed and upright. I wanted to cry about my messy house that is last on my "What can I manage today?" list. I wanted to complain about the crippling fatigue that comes in spells, and discouragement over not being able to do simple things that others take for granted.

Then I reminded myself that my life is also full of blessings:

- students who hug me for absolutely no reason; who come galloping into my classroom like they're going to Disney World; whose parents send meals when they know I'm struggling.
- co-workers who pray for me and make me homemade soup.
- a doctor friend who treats me for free.

- a boss who doesn't assign me to outdoor duties or anything too strenuous.
- friends and family who love me no matter what shape I'm in each day.

Suddenly I was smiling. *Other than my health,* I thought, *I have the perfect life for me. I love everything about it* . . . except for the Lyme disease. And maybe soon they'll come up with a definitive cure for it. Until then, I'll just keep working and napping and believing that tomorrow will be better.

The West Nile virus (WNV), which is now a world-wide pandemic, is carried by mosquitoes that have (usually) ingested blood from infected birds. It was first identified in the Western Hemisphere in 1999, in and around New York City, when seven patients presented with similar symptoms, and all of them died. The virus was detected soon afterward in Connecticut and New Jersey. The primary evidence was sick and dying crows, of which there were more than 10,000 found. It is thought that the first infected bird was brought into the U.S. illegally, but no one will ever know.

This virus has been around for an estimated 1,000 years, according to the report on Wikipedia.com, and may have even contributed to the early death of Alexander the Great. The virus was first isolated in the West Nile District of Uganda in 1937, but it was subsequently identified in Egypt (1942) and India (1953). A 1950 Egyptian study found that nine out of ten of those over forty years in age had WNV antibodies. In Israel in 1957, WNV was identified as a cause of severe human meningoencephalitis in the elderly. The disease was first noted in horses in Egypt and France in the early 1960s and found to be widespread in southern Europe, southwest Asia and Australia. Since the first North American cases in 1999, the virus has been reported throughout the United States, Canada, Mexico, the Caribbean, and Central America.[3]

With the current (late 2009) emphasis on H1N1 flu (swine flu), media attention on WNV has diminished. However, recent extensive studies of donated blood have shown that approximately 1 percent of Americans have antibodies to WNV, meaning they have been infected at one time or another. The CDC estimates that three million West Nile virus infections occurred between 1999 and 2008, representing a 100 percent increase over the prior five years. It doesn't take much interpolation to imagine the consequences of that kind of increase continuing for the next decade, for example, which is one reason that the CDC and other agencies worldwide are hard at work trying to develop a vaccine.

The good news, if there is any, about WNV, is that most infected persons survive. In fact, most infected persons do not even know they have been infected. According to a NIH/CDC release on the subject, "The majority of people—about 80 percent—who become infected with West Nile virus have no symptoms at all. Up to 20 percent may experience flu-like symptoms such as fever, headache and body aches or even nausea and vomiting. Only about one in 150 people will suffer severe illness, resulting in meningitis or encephalitis. People aged 50 and older are at higher risk for developing severe complications."[4]

The other good news is that for the insect-borne diseases (with CNS implications) that we've discussed in this chapter, prevention of infection can be the same for mosquitoes as it is for ticks. You can obtain some protection from your clothing—in fact, there are fine mesh suits available, complete with head nets, if you prefer not to use repellents. The most effective repellents contain DEET (N,N-diethyl-meta-toluamide), picaridin, oil of lemon eucalyptus, or IR 3535 (3-[N-Butyl-N-acetyl]-aminopropionic acid, ethyl ester), which is an active ingredient in at least one U.S.-made product. This repellent has been used in Europe for more than twenty years with no adverse side effects. Scientists have recently developed a new insect repellent that is made from oil of catmint. This has been shown to be effective with mosquitoes. No information is available on its effectiveness against ticks, but if you choose this one your cat may love you to death.

I (Dave) remember when I first used DEET. I just happened to take it with me on a spring bear hunt in Canada in 1974. Even though I have lived in the Upper Peninsula of Michigan, where the mosquitoes seem the size of hummingbirds, the ones in Canada ganged up on me in such numbers that they seemed like a bug-copter trying to carry me away, or perhaps like an army of "draculitos." Without that DEET, I might have returned to the States more or less bloodless.

Since then, DEET has come under much scrutiny, with some suggesting that it should be avoided due to possible long-term effects if it is ingested or over-applied to the skin, through which it is absorbed. However, DEET is rated as safe to use, even with children (not infants), as long as certain precautions are followed—see the CDC guidelines for comparison of insecticides and specific information on their use.[5] Other sites provide good information on the active ingredients in various products.[6] In general, the more "natural" products tend to provide less effective protection, especially when exposure to insects is prolonged.[7] So the choice, especially for parents trying to protect their children, is a true two-horned dilemma—on the one horn, you must decide how to reduce the risk of illness from insect bites; on the other, you must weigh the benefits versus the risks of the various insecticides available. Do the research, but do not do nothing to protect yourself and those you love when you do spend time outdoors.

| 29 |

Rearrange Your Living Space

The only difference between a rut and a grave is their dimensions.

—Ellen Glasgow, author[1]

It's easy to get into a rut and we do it for many reasons: it saves time, we're too busy, life is too fast-paced, and keeping things the same is just easier. We resist making changes because it's uncomfortable and staying in our comfort zone is often the best thing, or so we think. Most of us desire improvement, but we don't want to pay the price for it. But, did you know that making changes and getting out of your rut is good for your brain and will help you age more gracefully?

Scientists have known for several years that people who lead mentally stimulating lives build a "cognitive reserve" in their brains. Stimulating the brain generates new neurons and strengthens their connections, which results in better brain performance and a lower risk of developing Alzheimer's.[2]

The ideal situation is to build this reserve while we are young, but it is never too late to start. This means leading a healthy, active lifestyle *and* stimulating the brain with learning and doing new things. Making changes "alters motor pathways in the brain and encourages new cell growth," according to Barbara E. Riley, director of the Ohio Department of Aging.[3] Besides being good for your brain health, it just makes life more interesting.

One of the easiest ways of doing this is to change your living space. Even such simple things as planting new flowers in your yard, redecorating your kitchen, moving your furniture around, buying different color towels for the bathroom, and so on, will help stimulate those brain cells.

"I never change my furniture around or my decorating style," said Sue. "I move into a place, decorate it, and it stays that way until I move out. However, it does get boring after awhile. I have a friend who constantly changes her furniture, moving heavy pieces from room to room until she is satisfied. The only problem is, she is quickly dissatisfied and then goes at it again. Her family thinks it's funny—until they can't find something in a place where it used to be. She's like a woman Dave knows who changes her furniture so often that her husband has put the larger pieces on wheels! I recently bought new shelving for my living room and needed some things to go on the shelves. I actually found myself getting excited about rearranging old things and purchasing new things. The interesting thing is that once I got started, I wanted to make other changes and to do some things differently. I found that making a few changes lifted my spirits and I wanted to keep up the momentum. Hmm, let's see, maybe pink towels in the bathroom instead of green."

According to the Chinese, the goal in arranging your living space (or rearranging it), besides stimulating those brain cells, is to maximize feelings of safety and comfort, which will in turn positively affect your health, attitude, even your level of success.[4] Creating a pleasing visual space in your home by the way you have things arranged is good for your physical, emotional, and spiritual health.

How do you get started? Go room by room in your home and take inventory.

Remember, this does not have to be an expensive process, unless, of course, you have disposable income to make new purchases. Here are some ideas to get you started:

- Is the furniture arranged to maximize comfort, ease of movement, and to facilitate conversation and relationships with family and friends? Is your home office organized in a way to make your work easier? Is your kitchen arranged in a way that makes preparing a meal more of a pleasure than a chore? Making a few simple changes in furniture and room arrangement may make your life easier and more pleasant.

- How about the color scheme? Are the colors soothing and pleasing to the eye? Do you have a variety of colors, or are your rooms too monotone and perhaps boring?

- Add new colors with candles, plants, pictures, knick-knacks or other decorative ornaments, and some interesting books with brightly colored jackets on your tables and shelves—anything to add some color and interest to your living space. Tired of those towels in the bathroom? Changing the color can change the whole feel to the room.

- Check the lighting. Are there dark areas of your house, especially in the winter, that could use some better lighting? Are your curtains or window treatments blocking necessary sunlight? This is especially important if you live in an area where it remains dark much of the winter. Adding better lighting can help prevent Seasonal Affective Disorder (SAD), which will affect your mood, which, of course, helps your brain remain healthier.

- And, finally, is your home free from clutter? Nothing can ruin the mood of your home more than a lot of clutter and things out of place. Start by going room to room and disposing of what you don't need, finding new places for what you want to keep, and getting more organized. You'll find your mood and attitude will improve greatly by just taking this step.

Getting out of a rut and making changes is not easy. Finding your comfort zone and staying in it is much safer and easier sometimes. But, if you want to improve your life and your health, decide if you are worth it, then go for it.

| 30 |

Refuse to Retire

Don't simply retire from something; have something to retire to.

—Harry Emerson Fosdick, pastor[1]

Retirement is something you may be looking forward to and planning for, especially if you have spent many years in the workforce on the same job or in the same profession. You may have dreams of traveling, spending time with family and friends, getting your house and yard in order, or playing a few more rounds of golf a week. If you have saved and planned for your retirement, you may be looking at early retirement before age sixty-five.

Many of us remember our parents and grandparents and what it was like for them when they retired. Many were on a fixed income and didn't have discretionary money to do a lot of extra things. They spent the greater part of their days in front of the TV or sitting on the front porch. For most, there was no thought of working after retirement, so "retirement" became the time between work and when they died. Many of them also did not have access to leisure activities geared toward seniors that the elderly do today.

Times have changed and retirement is viewed differently by many. For those nearing retirement age, particularly Baby Boomers, retirement presents challenges. In a study done by AARP, of the seventy-six million Baby Boomers, the majority either can't or don't want to retire.[2] Leaving a job at fifty-five, sixty, or sixty-five and puttering around the house is becoming a thing of the past. Many people are delaying retirement or retiring differently. People live longer, have more energy, many are better off financially, and they want to stay active doing something they enjoy well into their golden years.[3]

I (Dave) see it this way. If the Bible is my guide for my life and my values, I have to admit that there is *nothing* in there about "retirement." Nobody retired, possibly because people didn't live long enough to qualify for social security, whatever that means. Moses kept going strong until the Lord took him home. The same is true for every other saint or role model in the entire Scriptures. Applying this to myself, at age sixty, I must ask: Why should I even want to "retire?" My life is full to the brim with creative activities that I hope will advance the cause of Christ. Whether it be editing a Christian medical magazine, or writing books like this one, or helping previously unpublished authors get published, or educating people regarding how to get their kids to eat healthier, I can't see a time now or in the future when I would want to back away from anything I'm doing.

A study completed by the Shell Oil Company and published in 2003 found that "People who retired early at age 55 had almost twice the risk of death compared to those who retired at age 60 or older or who continued working. The risk of early retirement was greater for men. Mortality improved with increasing age at retirement for people from both high and low socioeconomic groups. The health status of those who retired at 60, however, was similar to those who continued working at 60. Survival rates remained significantly greater for those who retired at 65 compared with those who retired at 55."[4]

Health factors may have contributed to early death of those who retired early, but mental health may have been a bigger factor. Working represents something to do, a connection with others, something with purpose and meaning, a place to belong. Work offers the opportunity to keep the brain stimulated and active, and helps stave off depression.

As you plan for retirement, look at what many people are doing and consider "reinventing" yourself. What does this look like? Kelly Carmichael Casey, a career counselor in Portland, Oregon, who works with Baby Boomers, says, "The expectations are that most of us need to continue to earn money after the traditional retirement age. Working has to have meaning and it has to feel as though it makes an impact in a positive way in the world."[5]

What does "reinventing" yourself look like in the real world?

• Start planning your dream job while you are still in your pre-retirement years. Jacquie was a social worker prior to her retirement, a career she'd had for many years. Knowing the income she'd need for retirement and planning that part-time job she would need to supplement her retirement income, she decided to do something she had always dreamed of doing—flower arranging.

"I love doing this, it's something I've always wanted to do, and it keeps my creative juices flowing," she said.

- Don't be afraid to take risks. If you've always wanted to work around boats but live where there is no water, consider moving to a place where your dreams just might happen. Or, consider starting your own business based on your experience, training, and interest. If you have years of business experience, consider consulting a few hours a week. If you taught school all your life, how about tutoring students who could use extra help?

- Volunteering is a wonderful way to keep yourself active, keep your mind stimulated, to feel that you are doing something with meaning and purpose and giving back. And very often, volunteering can turn into a real job. Russell and his wife retired to a small town where they became active in their church and community. A fitness buff, Russell spent hours at the local YMCA. Within a year he was the executive director.

- Planning should occur while you are still working and earning your regular income. Make a list of things you want to do, things you can do, the money you will need to earn, and what the ideal retirement would look like to you. With planning, you can make it happen.

Remember, a second career can be the best retirement, especially if you are doing something you love, something that keeps you physically active, mentally stimulated, socially connected, and spiritually rejuvenated.

| 31 |

Rejoice

Rejoice in the Lord always. I will say it again: Rejoice!
—the apostle Paul, from prison (Phil. 4:4, NIV)

Depending on which Bible translation you prefer, the word "rejoice" appears close to 300 times in the Bible. Its root concept is "joy," which is more than happiness, since happiness is connected to good happenings. Instead, joy is a much more settled attitude of the soul, contributing to stable emotions, a sound mind, and a strong will committed to living a life of love for God and one's fellow men.

One question worth asking is: Considering all we need to know in order to live well and finish well, why so much emphasis on joy and rejoicing? Answer: Like all divine directives, following His rules are in our best interest. Joy and rejoicing are a part of healthy living, the root of which is the Old English word *hælth*, i.e. wholeness in body, mind, and spirit.

We could stop there, except we want you to know that modern technology's non-invasive probing of the human brain is actually showing the positive effect that joy has on that organ. This being true, the data is worth considering even if one is not seeking a life of joy via the pathway of faith. For if sadness, depression, despair, and their associates cause disease in one's brain and joy and its associates create a context for optimal brain health, then it's a "no-brainer" for anyone interested in having the healthiest brain possible to find out all there is to know about this matter.

Thankfully, all there is to know on this matter is simple enough. When we're sad, angry, afraid, anxious, or addicted to some person, place, thing, or activity—our brain shows it when examined using SPECT (single photon emission computed tomography). SPECT, according to Wikipedia.com, is "a nuclear medicine tomographic imaging technique using gamma rays. It is very similar to conventional nuclear medicine planar imaging using a gamma camera. However, it is able to provide true 3D information."[1] Likewise, when we're content, hopeful, happy, and healthy (emotionally), the SPECT results show that, too. How it's done and how it's read are both book-length subjects, but one scientist investigating brain health using SPECT has written the book, *This Is Your Brain on Joy.*

Dr. Earl Henslin is a colleague of Dr. Daniel Amen, a pioneer in this field, whose SPECT scan work rules out bad wiring in the brain, either from birth or brain injury. These scans differ from regular imaging, in that they show the patient's brain while he or she is reacting, not just at rest. By interpreting the areas that "light up" in the patient's brain at certain times, doctors can get more input as to why some people are dysthymic (chronically mildly depressed or irritable), or have rage issues, or are obsessive-compulsives like the beloved Monk character of the TV show by the same name.

Interestingly enough, Henslin's patient SPECT scans reveal numerous details (not whether that particular brain is "normal," but which areas are more efficiently "wired" for a happy life). His brain scans reveal a sort of cerebral happy face if you concentrate on the illuminated sections of the brain while the patient is experiencing joy. Is this the Maker's sense of humor, to make our brains match our smiles when we are in the talons of joy?[2]

The researchers are looking at a variety of therapeutic options including psychotherapy, supplements, or prescription medications, sometimes all three, to see which can restore a particular patient to a happier state.

"What you choose to do, think about, surround yourself with, and put in your gullet make a difference," says Henslin. "It *all* matters to your experience of joy on this planet."[3] In addition, Henslin emphasizes that those who pray and meditate each day not only increase their peace and joy, but the calming effects of those two activities become more effective as time goes on, if they become a regular habit.[4]

In other words, even when times are tough, our choices about how and with whom to face adversity are perhaps the most important keys to rejoicing even in the sorrow. Susan knows this, firsthand:

First my husband left. Then my son got a job and moved out. I was okay with my empty nest, but I sometimes fought depression because, as a full-time homemaker in a high-stress marriage, I had been out of the workplace for over nineteen years. That was just long enough for my former career to disappear and my health to deteriorate. Interviews weren't producing a much-needed job and alimony was sporadic, but one day things got even worse. As suddenly as a tsunami, nausea left me immobilized, unable to even turn over in bed.

My friends offered help, and I assured them it was probably the flu. But it didn't go away. Was I neurotic? Imagining it? After three days, my doctor referred me to a gall bladder surgeon who scheduled surgery . . . five days off. I lay in bed for nearly a week, sipping water and dissolving crackers in my mouth, trying to be grateful for the inevitable weight loss (surely), wondering if all the stress in my life, my disastrous marriage particularly, had had a particularly toxic effect on my health. I was terrified. I had no money, no job, and I hoped my ex had remembered to pay for my minimal health insurance. He often "forgot." I had never felt more alone and powerless as I battled depressing thoughts about my past, present, and future.

All the negatives of my life were crowding out the good until I declared a sickly cease fire on them. Lying perfectly still, I recounted all the blessings of my life from childhood on. I would have liked to write them down, but I couldn't roll over to pick up a pen without severe nausea. And so I turned my bedroom TV to a show with nature scenes and praise music, and drifted in and out of sleep clutching my Bible. Operation day finally arrived and my son drove me to the hospital where I assured him I was fine.

A friend came and sat with me in the hospital outpatient waiting room for the ten hours before my surgery. I vaguely remembered patients coming and going; my pastor praying for me; my friend asking if I had told the doctors I was allergic to latex. (I hadn't, and that took another half-hour while they set up a latex-free operating room.) My next memory was waking up in the recovery room listening to the sound of fingernails being filed. "Nurse? I don't feel so good," I said. "Well waddaya expect? You just had surgery!" she grumbled, as she checked my IV.

If I hadn't been in such pain, or so groggy, I might have resented the nurse's tone, but I was right in the middle of another session of counting my blessings and afraid to break the momentum. It wasn't until I was in a *private* hospital room that I realized another unexpected blessing . . . being allergic to latex. It was hospital policy to separate out latex-sensitive patients in a private room unless they could find another latex-sensitive patient. And because of my wheat allergy, the food trays were prepared separately, and deliciously!

The IV with anti-nausea drugs and pain killers kicked in as I took stock of my world. Yes, I was still more or less indigent for all intents and purposes, and I had a drain coming out of my side into a bag pinned to my hospital gown. But the doctor had performed what everyone said was a near miracle of laparoscopic surgery since my gallbladder had assumed the shape of an alien life-form.

The doctor and anesthesiologist both agreed to settle for whatever the health insurance paid, and my three days in the hospital would give me a chance to rest and find out what cable TV was all about. I was so excited about not being nauseated, I stayed up all night watching old reruns of *Leave it to Beaver* . . . and praising God.

Three days later, I wavered a bit when the doctor hauled what felt like 100 yards of hose out of my abdomen minutes before a ninety-pound candy striper appeared with a wheelchair to roll me downstairs at the exact moment the fire alarm went off. I told the candy striper I hadn't come that far just to go up in flames, and directed him to the employee elevator, the only one still working. We made our escape off the floor and out the front door, past the fire trucks blocking the entrance. My son picked me up and delivered me to my friend, a nurse, who insisted I spend my first night in her guestroom and then fixed me a gourmet meal. Even with all the discomfort and holes in my body, my joy was limitless. I never again doubted that the Lord really does provide and He really does give joy (and even companionship) for the journey.

Obviously, the faith route can be a way to find joy in difficult times. Jesus, who was known as a man of sorrows, often spoke of joy. In one instance, He had just told His disciples of His coming death, which makes these words on that occasion all the more remarkable: "I have told you this," He said, "so that my joy may be in you and that your joy may be complete" (John 15:11 NIV).

Of course, each person must choose his or her own approach. Some prefer psychotherapy, medications, supplements, scented candles, soft music, or any number of non-religious means to try to build a bridge from sorrow to joy. Our recommendation is to use all the proven means available, including faith-related means, since with this approach you have nothing to lose and everything to gain, including something Jesus described as a joy that no one can take away.

| 32 |

Replay Good Times

To look backward for awhile is to refresh the eye, to restore it, and to render it the more fit for its prime function of looking forward.

—Margaret Fairless Barber, *The Roadmender*[1]

Have you ever been in the middle of doing something else when all of a sudden something in the present triggers a memory and you are beamed back into a past event that is as clear to you as though you were currently there? The feeling of nostalgia sweeps over you so intensely that you feel you are actually reliving the moment. It could be something as simple as a song you hear on the radio, a smell that reminds you of your grandmother's apple pie, a picture you see of the ocean at sunset that reminds you of a past romantic encounter, or something else equally as mesmerizing, and you're suddenly off on a trip down memory lane.

Nostalgic memories usually replay pleasant events, which is why nostalgia can help when you are lonely, depressed, psychologically vulnerable, or threatened. Nostalgia is almost always associated with positive emotions even when the trigger is something negative. The memory can even be bittersweet (happiness mixed with sadness), but the mind will juxtapose positive and negative elements to create redemption, moving the negative memory towards a positive one.

The term "nostalgia" was inspired by Homer's character, Odysseus, who, on his way home from the Trojan War, took respite for seven years with the beautiful sea nymph Calypso on the island of Ogygia. Calypso offered to make Odysseus immortal if he would stay with her. Love won out, however, because Odysseus pined for his wife, Penelope, and his home and longed to return to both. This longing for home became known as nostalgia from two Greek words, *nostos* for return and *algos* for pain. It is literally the "suffering due to the relentless yearning for the homeland."[2]

In their extensive research on nostalgia, scientists Sedikides, Widschut, Arndt, and Routledge state, "From the outset nostalgia was equated with homesickness. It was also considered a bad omen. In the 17th and 18th centuries nostalgia was regarded as a medical disease. Symptoms, including bouts of weeping, irregular heartbeat, and anorexia, were attributed to demons inhabiting the middle brain and other such phenomena. By the beginning of the 20th century, nostalgia was regarded as a psychiatric disorder. Symptoms included anxiety, sadness, and insomnia. By the late 20th century, nostalgia and homesickness parted ways. People regarded nostalgia as different from homesickness. Words such as *warm, old times, childhood*, and *yearning*, became more frequently associated with simple nostalgia rather than homesickness. Homesickness research focused on psychological problems, such as separation anxiety apparent when children leave the home environment, whereas nostalgia transcends social groups and age. Nostalgia is found cross-culturally and among well functioning adults and children and can refer to a variety of objects, not just a place of origin. The contemporary definition of nostalgia is a longing for one's past."[3]

The research of Sedikides and others focuses on the positive and potentially therapeutic aspects of nostalgia. Their research suggests that "Nostalgia can promote psychological health by producing positive feelings, higher self-esteem, and an increase in the feeling of being loved and protected by others. Nostalgia may boost optimism, spark inspiration, and foster creativity. Nostalgia also counteracts effects of loneliness, by increasing perceptions of social support. Loneliness can also trigger nostalgia and this has important implications for the elderly who are vulnerable to social isolation. Nostalgia may actually help them overcome feelings of loneliness."[4]

Nostalgia is about storytelling—stories created and stored as memories in your brain. You've probably noticed that each time you remember a positive past event, person, or place, the details are a little different. This is because a particular memory is not "retrieved," but is, in essence, re-created each time you recall it by a series of complex neural interactions. You've probably also noticed that as you grow older, the details of a particular event are fuzzier each time you recall it. This is again due to your brain re-creating, rather than retrieving, that particular story.[5]

Nostalgia provides a link between our past and present stories. By providing a positive view of the past, nostalgia serves to bring a greater sense of constructive continuity and meaning to our lives. While day-to-day living can become tedious and sometimes depressing, a positive look back at our own journey can change that perspective and add new meaning to what we are doing today.[6]

Nostalgia can create feelings of connection, because it isn't just about ourselves, but is also about our relationships with others. This creates a social context that helps us feel close to others who are important to us, and to feel that we are important to them, too.

Nostalgia can also help us place ourselves in the context of our community and its history—of course this assumes that we still live in or near the community of our upbringing. Visiting local museums is a great place to remember the history of our town, still being written through us. Old photographs help us see what our town (and the people in it) looked like "back in the olden days" when people walked to work, went to church, wore their Easter bonnets in the Easter Parade, and made their own clothes instead of paying someone a half-world away to do that. Another good source for nostalgic local information or photos is your local library, which is likely to have a section devoted to local history. If you engage with your family in these and similar activities, then your kids will never be wandering around wondering who they are or, as some would put it, "trying to find themselves." One of the more humorous stories that I (Dave) have heard about this involved a youth minister's friend, who picked up one such wanderer one day. The fellow was hitchhiking to who knows where, and in the midst of the whole rather esoteric conversation, admitted that he was just trying to find himself. The driver pulled into a mall parking lot, took the hitchhiker to the big map in the middle of the mall, where there was a star marking the spot where they were standing. The driver touched the spot, and said, "You're here, man," and left the disoriented fellow to figure it out for himself.

Scrapbooking is another way to preserve your most precious memories, for yourself and posterity. And with the advent of the digital age, a number of new methods exist that make it much easier to achieve a similar effect, as in "scrapbooking" online, or creating screensavers or a slideshow of your favorite photos, including nostalgic ones, on your computer screen whenever it's turned on.

Recently, my wife and I (Dave) lost our very dear friend and companion, Brownie (an English springer spaniel) after nearly ten years of loving and rubbing, swimming and sharing our bed at night, even when we were camping. As a way of remembering him and the joy he brought us, we purchased a digital photo frame, which is comprised of a memory chip and a monitor-like display that just keeps sorting through our favorites of the nearly 1,000 photos we had preserved—digital cameras make it a lot easier, for sure. At first, this was hard to watch, but now we feel more joy that we had him, if only for a little while, than regret or sadness that he couldn't stay with us longer.

Another high-tech nostalgia helper is called a "voice quilt." My sister is the family historian, having tracked our roots back several generations (that's not only nostalgic but educational). For our parents' eightieth birthdays, she invited a host of family and friends to contribute to a voice quilt for each of them. The process is simple, and the product is both inspired and inspiring. Potential participants receive a telephone number to call, where they can record their greeting. Many shared greetings began with "remember when." In the process of listening to these, a myriad of faded memories resurfaced, and the neurological connections were renewed. For all of us, it was like a journey back in time, but the great thing about it was that not only did the whole process renew old memories, it developed new ones that we shared together as we listened to the past, in the present. Now that's a synaptic event, for sure.

So however you practice your own nostalgic moments, keep in mind that there really is something to the old adage, "Nostalgia ain't what it used to be." Nope. It's better!

| 33 |

Resolve Damaging Emotions

The sky is falling! The sky is falling!

—Chicken Little

Emotions such as worry, fear, guilt, anxiety, and anger are hazardous to your health. Scientists have known for years that these and other emotions can cause a myriad of physical problems, and are the culprits behind many mental and emotional problems, such as depression, anxiety, and panic disorders.

In recent years studies have shown just how damaging these emotions can be to your brain health, and the research is showing that if you want your brain to be happy, you need to be happy, too. One of the ways to be happy is to take control of your emotions instead of allowing them to control you.

New York neuroscientist Joseph Ledoux has studied how the brain processes emotions, especially fear. He describes

174

the "amygdala, the almond-shaped brain structure that interprets emotion, as 'the hub in the brain's wheel of fear.' When the amygdala is stimulated, there is an outpouring of stress hormones, causing a state of hyper-vigilance. The amygdala processes the primitive emotions of fear, hate, love, bravery, and anger—all neighbors in the deep limbic brain. When the amygdala malfunctions, a mood disorder, or state of uncontrollable apprehension results." The amygdala, then, is an important component of the circuit that regulates negative emotion.[1]

Not only does the amygdala process current fearful circumstances, but in collaboration with other parts of the brain, it helps us remember *past* fearful memories. For example, if you were abandoned by someone important to you as a child, you may have difficulty forming close relationships as an adult because of your fear that that person or persons may leave you also. Your brain's thalamus alerts your amygdala, which triggers the fearful memory, and your body goes into overdrive. According to Joseph Ledoux, this is a warning system malfunction, because it is alerting you to danger that may no longer threaten you.[2]

This is further explained by Timothy Stokes, PhD. The amygdala "plays a central role in the storage of 'emotion memories'—unconscious memories of past hurts: times, especially in childhood, when we were painfully rejected, physically harmed, humiliated, helplessly frustrated, and so on. An emotion memory is recalled unconsciously. These memories are very durable and without intervention they may last a long time—even a lifetime. These emotion memories create feelings that are not appropriate to our immediate situation. When an emotion memory is active, we make distorted assumptions about our current situation. Hormones inhibit the reality-testing part of our brain, leading us to believe and even defend a distorted view of what is going on."[3] Unfortunately, these problems are being generated by brains that are functioning exactly as they were designed to function.

Fear is the underlying and primary emotion for much of what we feel and how we behave. It's part of our genetic makeup and functions to keep us safe in dangerous situations. You may be familiar with the "Fight or Flight" response to stimuli. When confronted with a situation that we are unfamiliar with or afraid of, all of our bodily systems are sent into a hyper state of alertness. The result is an outpouring of hormones, including adrenaline, followed by the hormone cortisol. This helps us to quickly assess the situation as one we either need to flee or fight. If we hear a strange noise in our home at night, our senses shift into alert mode and we will either go investigate or decide that it's nothing. We can grab our .38 Special or calm down.[4]

When there is something stressful or fearful that we need to deal with, we have an adrenaline rush. The problem comes when stress becomes constant, rather than transitory. The result is worry, anxiety, and even panic. Panic is a heightened state of anxiety. Anxiety, distress, panic, and fear are closely related negative emotional states associated with physical or psychological harm. Anxiety is characterized by the anticipation of being harmed in the future, whereas fear is characterized as the anticipation of being harmed in the present. Distress is characterized by the awareness of being harmed at this particular moment. All of these can diffuse into one harmful emotional state or another.

What causes fear, worry, anxiety, panic, and other harmful emotions? Almost anything and everything can contribute. In a society where we have just about everything we need at our fingertips, where we are relatively healthy and safe, and where we have opportunities that past generations never imagined, we still worry and fret that we won't have enough, that we will catch the latest disease, and a myriad of other things. Many of us have "Chicken Little Syndrome" like that fairy tale character who thought the sky was falling and there was no hope for the future.

Bob was a consummate worrier. He worried about his job, being able to care for his family, having enough money to pay his bills, his health, and just about everything else. A child of the Depression, he grew up without enough and this mindset stayed with him the rest of his life. Even after receiving a rather large inheritance and investing it wisely, he worried about outliving his savings. His wife told him not to worry, that God would take care of them. Bob did without many comforts through the years because of his fear that he wouldn't have enough. He didn't outlive his savings and left his widow comfortable, although not wealthy. She has now picked up his mantle of worry and is concerned that she will outlive her savings, although she is very frugal and has done well. She is learning, however, that all of this worry and fear could shorten her life and she is doing some of the things she always wanted to do, such as travel, trusting that God will indeed provide—just as He always has.

We know that fear, worry, and anxiety are bad for our health. Is it really possible to decrease negative effects of that little part of our brain, the amygdala, and keep those necessary, but potentially damaging, hormones from controlling us? There are ways of reducing fear and inhibiting the fear response. Your fear and anxiety are caused by, in large part, your own thoughts and self-talk. It is important to stop those thoughts before they get out of control. Visualize a stop sign and put it in your mind when you start to go down a rabbit trail of negative emotion. Tell yourself that you won't go there because the trail leads to a place you don't want to go. Many have also overcome anxiety by seeing a pastor or counselor trained to deal with this problem. Talking to someone provides social interaction, which also results in a healthy and happy brain.

Your thoughts are under *your* control. It's as easy to tell yourself the truth as it is to believe a lie. It takes practice to undo the negative thought patterns that lead to fear, worry, anxiety, and so forth, but you'll be a happier and healthier person if you do, and you'll probably live longer too.

| 34 |

Stay Focused

A well-orchestrated "executive brain" knows its priorities.

—Adam J. Cox, PhD[1]

The most important functions that our brain performs are the ones that make us who we are, wielding executive control and mediating our ability to focus in spite of life's distractions. The brain's CEO areas not only help us focus but also enable us to consciously study and retain information and behave appropriately as settings change. These areas of the brain are primarily located in the prefrontal cortex and are important because they are often tied to cognitive decline in aging. Our ability to memorize, plan, schedule, and juggle multiple tasks has its roots here. Recent studies are showing that these areas of the aging brain, with training, can end up reacting pretty much the same as in younger adults.

New research at the University of Illinois at Urbana-Champaign shows that brain training reignites key areas, boosting performance. Participants in this study were thirty-two men and women, ages fifty-five to eighty, and thirty-one younger adults. They were divided into control and experimental groups and run through a battery of brain testing. Before and after results showed significant improvement in the prefrontal cortex area in both the old and the young. Researchers commented that the old and young react in very much the same way with this type of training, thus countering aging factors.[2] So we really are never too old to learn new skills.

In addition to brain training, researchers continue to report that aerobic exercise can prevent and possibly even reverse decline in these key areas of "executive control." The exercise must be strenuous enough to make a person slightly "breathless" and should be continued for at least thirty minutes (but should never be started without an okay from your physician). This type of exercise can not only improve the way the brain functions, but it also increases the volume of brain tissue. It has been shown that after only about six months of aerobic exercise people with age-related brain decline show evidence of their brain "plasticity" or capacity growing and developing.[3]

A crucial role of our brain's CEO is to trigger safe behavior and keep us from harm. This area of the brain seems to be more concerned about the consequences of our actions than how hard they are to produce. One theory is that our CEO is constantly monitoring itself so that appropriate actions or change of direction can take place. "Ability to realistically appraise our behavior at all times is especially important as we face dangerous or technically difficult situations. Executive functions are often invoked when it is necessary to override responses that may otherwise be automatically elicited by stimuli in the external environment."[4]

Anyone who has ever been on a diet is familiar with this struggle. You see a big piece of apple pie and you want it. Your CEO clicks in and tries to inhibit this automatic response! There can be a bit of a tug-of-war. One way researchers can test executive function control is by using flash cards that have the names of colors printed on them but in different ink colors. For instance the word purple may be printed in green ink. This presents our CEO with a dilemma. If asked to say what you see, your automatic response would be to say the word, "purple." But you would have to override the automatic response when asked to look at the card and name the color in which the word is printed. Or how about when you move to a new neighborhood and find you have automatically driven home to the old house? Or, much more serious, you are driving and a text comes in from your best friend and you decide to focus on reading and answering it?

Texting has become an enormously popular way of communicating, but with the convenience comes grave danger if attempted while driving. There are numerous fatal accidents attributed to texting, like the seventeen-year-old student from Eureka, Illinois, who was killed when she drove off the road while sending a message to her friends. Then there was the tragic train crash that occurred in California in 2009 when the train engineer was involved with sending and receiving text messages seconds before he missed a red light and collided head on with a freight train; needlessly killing twenty-five people. Several other reports have confirmed the risk of this dangerous trend. The Virginia Tech Transportation Institute found that when drivers of heavy trucks texted, their collision risk was twenty-three times greater than when not texting. Another report by *Car and Driver* magazine found that texting while driving is more dangerous than driving under the influence of alcohol.[5] Clearly something must be done to protect the public and educate all drivers about this dangerous act.

One bright spot is the tech companies who are concerned, often for personal reasons, about these dangers associated with their high tech phones. Matt Howard, a co-founder of *Zoomsafer*, was rattled when he barely missed hitting his neighbor's son while texting. He immediately began looking for an application for his Blackberry that would prevent this from happening again and to his surprise could find nothing. *Zoomsafer* is now scheduled to become available in the very near future, followed by other applications by firms who are working on additional text prevention devices for use while driving.

Texting while driving leads to increased distraction behind the wheel. In 2006, Liberty Mutual Insurance Group conducted a survey with more than 900 teens from over twenty-six high schools nationwide. The results showed that 37 percent of students found texting to be "very" or "extremely" distracting. A study by the AAA discovered that 46 percent of teens admitted to being distracted behind the wheel due to texting.

A 2009 experiment with *Car and Driver* magazine editor Eddie Alterman that took place at a deserted air strip showed that texting while driving had a greater impact on safety than driving drunk. While legally drunk, Alterman's stopping distance from 70 miles per hour increased by four feet; by contrast, reading an e-mail added thirty-six feet, and sending a text added seventy feet.[6] As you would expect, when attention is being diverted to texting, the brain's CEO is occupied and unable to detect dangerous but subtle changes. For instance, if we are paying close attention while at the wheel, we will notice that the light is about to change or there is a car approaching rapidly from the rear, or a car on the left is making slight movements toward our lane, or a small child is running toward the street. Failure to detect hazards and respond quickly increases stopping time by three car lengths. This distance can make the difference between causing or avoiding an accident and between fatal and non-fatal consequences. Losing focus while driving also makes the driver unable to maintain consistent safe distance from other cars as well as stay in their own lane. Talking on the cell phone while driving can also be dangerous and is why cell phone use while driving is now banned in a number of states. But as dangerous as cell phone use is, texting is far worse—especially if you are composing and sending a text.

Possessing the ability to maintain executive control is a valuable asset and one we must preserve and protect as we age. Adam J. Cox has written a book geared to helping children maintain executive control, but his principles can be applied to all ages. He lists the following "eight pillars of executive control":

Initiation—being able to organize one's thoughts and begin a task

Flexibility—learning to adapt by shifting focus and pace as situations change

Attention—focusing well enough to learn important information and block distraction

Organization–being able to manage your space

Planning—being able to manage time and clarify priorities

Working Memory—the ability to retain information long enough to store it in long-term memory

Self-Awareness—knowing yourself and how others see you

Regulating Emotions—expressing feelings appropriately so as not to over-react[7]

Keep these eight pillars in mind as you seek to increase your focus and stay sharp mentally. Improve them, one by one, and you'll be happier, healthier, and safer in the long run.

| 35 |

Stay Socially Active

The value of a relationship is in direct proportion to the time that you invest in the relationship.

—Brian Tracy, motivational speaker[1]

Researchers have known for many years that having good social networks is good for your physical, mental, emotional, and spiritual well-being. But recent studies are also finding that supportive relationships can be advantageous to your brain health as well. The amount of contact you have with others is a good indication as to how well you will maintain sharp mental capabilities as you age.

AARP reports, "A major public-health study involving more than 116,000 participants found that people with strong relationships had less mental decline and lived more active, pain-free lives without physical limitations. Other studies suggest that people with the most limited social connections

185

are twice as likely to die over a given period than those with the widest social networks. Many experts believe that social isolation may create a chronically stressful condition that accelerates aging."[2]

Loners don't age as well as those who keep socially active. Michael Merzenich, PhD, a neurobiologist at the University of California, San Francisco, said, "As soon as you become captive in your room or your chair, you've got a problem. You become removed from the possibilities for excitement, for learning, and for engaging your brain with fun and surprise. Your brain needs you to get out and have those 1,000 daily surprises."[3]

It's easier to develop and maintain relationships when you're younger and more active. Friendships often develop over common interests and activities such as work, school, church, children, hobbies, sports, and so on. Simple activities, such as having a cup of coffee with a friend, can help to dispel stress, unhappiness, depression, loneliness, and a host of other mental and emotional issues detrimental to your health.

However, in today's fast-paced, overly busy society, maintaining social connections is something that has to be actively pursued and worked at. Research shows that over the last twenty years there has been an increase in social isolation in America. This is, in part, due to long work hours and hours spent surfing the internet, versus spending at least some of that time with friends, in person.[4] It is also related to the increased mobility of Americans due to job change and other factors, which make it difficult to maintain relationships and to develop new ones.

Older people often lead solitary lives because family and friends are no longer living close by. More and more people are opting to retire in a warmer climate, which often means leaving close relationships behind. Older adults also face the loss of marriage partners and other close relationships through death. There is a general decline in overall health, especially in older adults, after the death of a life partner. It is especially important for this age group to maintain and develop relationships and activities that help keep them connected, mentally alert, and physically healthy. This is easier for them if they are involved in senior centers, church groups, or other community organizations that provide opportunities for meaningful and active lifestyles.

Margaret is eighty-five, living on her own after the death of her husband of fifty-nine years. She has chosen to remain in her own home because financially that makes the best sense. Because of declining health and a lack of mobility, she has found it difficult to remain socially connected and, at first, didn't want to. "After Bob died, I stayed by myself a lot and didn't really see anyone unless they came to see me," she said. "However, I found that my mental sharpness was slipping in small ways, such as forgetting to turn off the oven, and I realized that I needed to be around other people and get out and do things. I make sure that I get out and spend time with friends at least once a week and stay connected by telephone. This has helped keep me alert. I plan on joining a seniors' Bible study."

A report posted at www.fitbrains.com says that "identifying opportunities for socialization in your community and combining that with your own innate talents can foster an enriched environment for your brain health. Research suggests a potentially important health role for maintaining socialization across the lifespan. The activities a person engages in throughout their life may have an impact upon their brain health and perhaps affect their vulnerability to neurodegenerative disease.

"Social engagement may challenge people to communicate effectively and to participate in complex social interactions. Social engagement fosters a dynamic, novel environment. It also requires a commitment to community and family that may promote a sense of belonging and purpose. There is also an immediate social network fostered by social engagement that can assist in many ways including emotional support.

"Research has explored the relationship between the amount and type of activity, and the risk for dementia. Findings indicate that older persons with five or six social ties are significantly less likely to demonstrate cognitive decline compared to those who had no social ties.

"Developing strong family ties and friendships is not a given nor is it easy. However, as part of the lifestyle for a healthy brain the importance of nurturing our relationships cannot be underestimated. Our ability to continually develop relations and sustain them across the lifespan represents a real proactive, health promoting behavior."[5]

Here are a few ideas to help you make new friends and keep your old friends:

- Pursue social activities—join a club, take a class, join a gym, get involved at your church and in your community, develop a hobby that gets you involved with others, volunteer, travel with friends, learn to play a musical instrument, and so on. There are hundreds of ways to get out there and get connected with others.
- Remain physically active—take a walk, take your dog to the dog park, take up golf or tennis, take a yoga class, learn to gourmet cook, join a biking or hiking club, anything that keeps your body moving. Again, the ideas and opportunities are limitless.

- Cultivate your friends—stay in touch, accept invites to social activities, issue invites, visit and take coffee and muffins to a friend who is having difficulties, send notes, make phone calls, and use any other means you can think of to keep those existing relationships alive and well.

- Maintain friendships with a positive outlook and attitude—ditch the negativity, gossip, and self-absorption. Learn to listen and be interested in what others have to say, learn what they are up to, and find ways to show your love and gratitude for their friendship. You'll be happier and healthier, and so will they.

| 36 |

Stop Killing Your Brain with Your Fork

Don't dig your grave with knife and fork.

—Old English Proverb

Most of us try to be quite focused on ways to grow more neurons and stay mentally sharp as we age. We do our crossword puzzles or Sudoku and try to stay active and involved with positive people. But we may be missing one very important safeguard that presents hazards every single day as we pick up a fork. The food we are feeding our brain could become its assassin.

There are two ways that unhealthy foods can hijack our brain. One way harms us in the same manner that nicotine robs our neurons—by clogging arteries and restricting blood flow. This reduces the levels of oxygen and healthy nutrients reaching our neurotransmitters. The second way foods make the "bad for the brain" list is by causing a roller coaster or crash and burn effect in our body. These foods not only harm the brain but also can cause wild mood swings and unproductive behavior as well as obesity.

Dr. David Kessler, former FDA chief, calls the "culprit foods 'layered and loaded' with combinations of fat, sugar, and salt—and often so processed that you don't even have to chew much."[1] Neuroscientists continue to report that foods laden with fat/sugar combinations turn on the brain's dopamine pathway. This area is the pleasure center of the brain and is the very same place that fuels people's addiction to alcohol or drugs. It has even been reported recently that saturated bad fats can be a causative factor in Alzheimer's disease by damaging the blood vessel lining of the brain just as it does in the heart.[2] Additionally, an increasing number of neuroscientists believe that the wide variety of "neurotoxins" in our environment and our food are having a detrimental effect on health in general and brain health in particular. The list of these toxic substances is long, but includes certain artificial sweeteners and monosodium glutamate, a common food additive.[3]

Dr. Kessler, who admits to being a fellow sufferer, has gathered researchers to find reasons why some people have such a hard time eating a healthy diet. He calls those who have great difficulty controlling what they eat "conditioned hyper eaters." Dr. Kessler found in a major study that this population of people reports feeling a loss of control over food and is preoccupied by food. He estimates that up to seventy million people have some degree of conditioned hyper eating.[4] Dr. Kessler's new book, *The End of Overeating*, explains his strategies to overcome these brain and body damaging tendencies.

It's Monday, 10 a.m. and "Alex Everyman"[5] is seeing his doctor for his annual physical. Alex is forty-two, 5'9" tall, and weighs 230 pounds. His doctor explains that, with each passing year, Alex is becoming more at risk for a variety of chronic illnesses. Every time Alex has come in for his physical in the past five years, he has gained a few more pounds and lost a little more hair. And each time his doctor has suggested that Alex should lose some weight by getting more exercise and changing his diet. This time, however, the doctor asks him to return in a week, with a daily diet diary of everything he eats or drinks in the next seven days.

The following Monday Alex reluctantly returns with his food diary and watches his doctor frown as he looks over the list of high-calorie meals. Then he says, "Thanks for your honesty, Alex, but you remind me of someone, an old friend . . . one of my classmates in med school. He lived to eat, it seemed, and to pretend his weight was not an issue, he would refer to himself as 'the poster boy for *Bon Appétit*.'"

"Really," Alex replies. "I can identify with that, for sure. How's he doing today?"

"He had a heart attack and died when he was forty-seven." The doctor pauses for emphasis, then adds, "We've talked about your cardiovascular risks before, but research is now showing that obesity affects the brain, too. Here is an article that came out recently. This is what it says: 'a new study finds obese people have 8 percent less brain tissue than normal-weight individuals. Their brains look 16 years older than the brains of lean individuals. Those classified as overweight have 4 percent less brain tissue and their brains appear to have aged prematurely by 8 years.'[6] What it means is that if you do grow old, and you don't get the weight under control, you'll also be at risk for Alzheimer's, since your BMI right now is 32.5 and 30 or more is the definition of obesity."[7]

As dangerous as saturated fat is in our food, sugary treats vie for first place among brain-damaging assassins. Dr. Larry

McCleary has long been prodding us to eat healthy for the sake of our body and brain. He explains the stealth method that sugar and processed flour use to rob us of brainpower. Dr. McCleary refers to the balance our bodies seek, by design, as the "Goldilocks Principle," named after the children's story of *Goldilocks and the Three Bears* in which Goldilocks is looking for things to be "just right" and does not want her porridge too hot or too cold, or her bed too soft or too hard. Dr. McCleary states that "neurons have similar needs when it comes to glucose and insulin levels. . . . the major fuel the brain burns is sugar, or more precisely glucose."[8]

Proper sugars (glucose), like good fats, are vital to the functioning of our brain, and the brain grabs onto 20 percent of the carbohydrates that we consume. Problems arise when we ingest sugar and *simple* carbohydrates in the wrong amounts and at the wrong times. If the timing and content is off we drag our body and brain onto a roller coaster for a wild ride throughout the day. Bad brain foods cause our blood sugar levels to shoot up temporarily, which puts stress on the pancreas and triggers a powerful rush of insulin to be released into our bloodstream. This overabundance of insulin leads to plummeting blood sugar levels along with a release of hormones manufactured in the adrenal glands, cortisol and epinephrine. High levels of these hormones in turn have the potential to kill brain cells and even stress the liver. This roller coaster effect causes us to shift from feeling happy and energetic while "high" on glucose to becoming sleepy, irritable, unfocused, or even agitated—not a good way to have a productive day! To protect themselves from these highs and lows, neurons and other cells eventually become *resistant* to the action of the insulin. This can lead to diabetes.

What your body and brain crave is a consistent flow of the "just right" amount and type of fuel throughout the day to give a consistent blood glucose level. Eating good brain foods that are known as high glycemic index foods will give your brain the boost it needs to keep your memory and neurotransmitters humming along at productive levels. Some of the stars are: Omega-3s, fruits, veggies, berries, whole grains, and spices. For more information on "good brain foods" see our chapter "Feed Your Neurons Well." And, *please* do everything you can to stop killing your brain with your fork. After all, there are much faster ways to leave this far-too-sweet place behind, but not too many work more efficiently.

| 37 |

Teach Your Brain to Tango

There are short-cuts to happiness, and dancing is one of them.

—Vicki Baum[1]

The hippocampus is central to learning and memory. It is also connected to the regions of the brain where executive functions take place, such as planning, problem solving, and multi-tasking. So it is not surprising that so many studies focus on this section of the brain when exploring age-related memory loss and cognitive decline. It has been known for some time that the hippocampus typically shrinks as we grow older. Recent studies have revealed some very good news: the health of our hippocampus is not fatalistically tied to a trajectory of decay going from our youthful endowment (its zenith) and leading to age-related deterioration (its nadir). The health of your hippocampus is within your own domain of influence. Here are some new discoveries relating to this vital part of the brain.

Exercise and fitness can increase the number of brain cells in the hippocampus. Researchers from the University of Illinois and the University of Pittsburgh measured the cardiorespiratory fitness of 165 adults (109 of them female) between fifty-nine and eighty-one years of age.[2] There was a strong correlation between fitness and hippocampus size. They tested the participants' spatial reasoning and found a significant association between an individual's physical fitness and his or her performance on certain spatial memory tests. "The higher fit people have a bigger hippocampus, and the people that have more tissue in the hippocampus have a better spatial memory," said University of Indiana psychology professor Art Kramer, who co-led the study with University of Pittsburgh psychology professor Kirk Erickson. ". . . [W]e see there is this significant and substantial relationship between how fit you are and how good your memory is, or at least a certain kind of memory, a certain kind of memory that we need all the time,"[3] Kramer said.

Exercise that involves memorizing forms is also shown to improve hippocampus function. In a three-year study of forty-two healthy and active seniors, a group that engaged in Tai Chi was compared with a healthy and active control group of non-Tai Chi practitioners. The Tai Chi group demonstrated significantly better eye-hand coordination skills, measured in numerous ways.[4] The memorization and execution of forms, which is central to Tai Chi, is often absent in other forms of exercise and even many sports.

Helen is in her late seventies. Years ago she joined a seniors group for dancing. They meet every week at the local synagogue and dance for ninety minutes with only a short break to rehydrate. In her dancing group, they do mostly line dancing, because many come unaccompanied. They learn a new dance every couple of weeks. There is a mix of dances, because the dancers are not all of equal health, balance, or vitality. Many of the dances are quite vigorous. She only sits down when the dance has become too vigorous and there has been a lot of turning and spinning. She proudly says that she almost never sits down.

From a brain health perspective, dancing is great activity. It can provide vigorous exercise, which by itself is one strategy for promoting brain health and cognition.[5] And learning new dance steps requires a type of learning known as learning for recall, which is important for brain health. Dancing is also a very social activity. Helen really enjoys her group of friends, all of whom she met through dancing. This keeps her connected. But what really keeps Helen returning week after week is that dancing is fun! Having fun is a great antidote for seasonal malaise and depression, both of which tear down rather than build up your brain.

Recent research indicates that the brain benefits from observing dance nearly as much as from the physical experience of dancing itself. Published by the Dana Foundation for Brain Research[6] in 2008, and available for download, the 146-page document *Learning, Arts, and the Brain*, was the result of three years of research by cognitive neuroscientists from seven leading universities across the United States.

"Dance and the Brain," is a section from this report. The section authors state, "[O]ur studies concerned the mechanisms that allow us to learn to dance, and the concurrent learning-related changes in the brain. Prior behavioral research on observational learning suggests that physical and observational learning share many common features. Neuroimaging research on action observation has identified brain regions, including premotor, inferior parietal, and temporal regions, that are similarly active when performing actions and when watching others perform the same actions. The present study investigated the sensitivity of this 'action observation network' (AON) to learning that is based on observation, compared to physical rehearsal.

"Participants were trained for five consecutive days on dance sequences that were set to music videos in a popular video game context. They spent half of daily training physically rehearsing one set of sequences, and the other half passively watching a different set of sequences. Participants were scanned with fMRI (functional magnetic resonance imaging) prior to, and immediately following, the week of training.

"Results indicate that premotor and parietal components of the AON responded more to trained, relative to untrained, dance sequences. These results suggest that activity in these brain regions represents the neural resonance between observed and embodied actions. Viewing dance sequences that were only watched (and not danced) also was associated with significant activity in the brain's premotor areas, inferior parietal lobule, and basal ganglia."[7]

So dance or learn to dance, but when you can't, watch one of the various dance competitions on TV, or get out a dance video—they're available from A to Z, or perhaps we should say, from Bachata to Waltz, and whatever else suits your taste, including Ballroom, Carolina Shag, Cha Cha, Disco, Foxtrot, Hustle, Merengue, Riverdance, Rumba, Salsa, Slow Dancing, Swing, Tango, or Texas Two Step. Or enjoy a dancing movie like *Footloose*, or one of the ten movies featuring the unmatchable grace of Fred Astaire and Ginger Rogers. Speaking for myself (Dave), I never cease to marvel when I watch Michael Flatley's "Feet of Flames." Every time I see it, my brain explodes.

| 38 |

Tune In to Your Senses

When you start using senses you've neglected, your reward is to see the world with completely fresh eyes.

—Barbara Sher, career counselor, author[1]

Imagine going through life without the ability to see the beauty around you, taste your favorite foods, smell your world after a spring rain, touch those you love, or to hear your favorite sounds. If you didn't have your senses, your world would be a very boring, and even unsafe, place.

Those of us who have our senses in working order, that is the senses of sight, taste, smell, touch, hearing, and often forgotten number six, proprioception, tend to take them for granted until they become less acute as we age. Scientists have long known that as we grow older the way our senses are able to give us information about our world changes. These changes happen slowly over the course of aging so that we often don't notice subtle decreases, especially with the senses of smell, taste, and touch. The most dramatic changes occur with vision and hearing.

Our senses receive information from the environment, such as light and sound vibrations. Receptors in our sense organs convert this information into nerve impulses which are then carried to the brain. Our brains interpret these impulses into the correct sensation. We require a certain amount of stimulation before a sensation is perceived. This is a minimum level or a "threshold." Aging increases the threshold so that the amount of sensory input necessary to be aware of the sensation becomes greater.[2]

The following is a brief description of your six senses, how they change as you age, and what you can do to help keep them young. In any of these areas try inhibiting one sense for a task and engaging another, such as eating a meal blindfolded or lighting candles while you eat. This helps keep your brain active.

Hearing: Your ears have two jobs—hearing and helping you to maintain balance. As you age, your ear structures deteriorate. The eardrum may thicken and the inner ear bones and other structures are affected. It often becomes more difficult to maintain balance. There may be hearing loss, especially for high-frequency sounds. The sharpness of hearing starts declining after the age of fifty. Your brain may have a decreased ability to process sounds into meaningful information. Some people with significant hearing loss may require hearing aids. Mike was a singer in a band in his youth and worship leader at his church for many years. The loud music took its toll on his hearing and he now requires a hearing aid and is less able to distinguish the sounds of the music he previously enjoyed.[3]

What can you do? Turn down the music, but keep listening. Music is a great brain stimulant. Combining sensory stimulation helps build new associations between areas of the brain. Try watching a sport in which you know the rules and the meaning of the referee's or umpire's signals on TV with the volume muted, and turn the radio on tuned to something else, to give your brain a good workout. For example, you might watch *Monday Night Football* to a CD of waltzes by Johann Strauss II.[4]

Vision: Age-related changes in vision can occur as early as your thirties. Fewer tears will be produced and your eyes will be drier. As you age the sharpness of your vision gradually declines and cataracts may begin to form. There are also changes in response to darkness or bright light, thus the inability of some seniors to drive at night. Martha is eighty-six and can still drive herself around during the day, but had to curtail her night driving many years ago. This has meant a loss of independence and social activity for her. Corrective eyewear will help with most of the problems you incur as you age. Your peripheral vision will decrease, making it harder to drive and do other activities you've enjoyed. In addition, your ability to distinguish colors decreases. It becomes harder to distinguish blues and greens than reds and yellow.[5] Mary's creative solution to distinguishing between what had become lookalike clothing (black and navy blue) was to sew a special tag into the navy clothing.

What can you do? Have a yearly eye exam to make sure that any deterioration of vision is due to normal aging. Keep your eyes active with reading and other activities that help keep your vision sharp and stimulate your brain.

Taste and Smell: The senses of taste and smell are closely related. Most taste comes from odors. As well as providing enjoyment, these senses alert us to dangers such as spoiled food, hazardous materials, and smoke. You have approximately 9,000 taste buds. Their number starts decreasing around the age of forty to fifty in women and fifty to sixty in men. Sensitivity to salty, sweet, bitter, and sour tastes doesn't decrease until after age sixty. The sense of smell usually doesn't diminish until after age seventy. Some studies have indicated that normal aging produces very little change in taste and smell. Rather, these changes may be due to diseases, smoking, and other environmental factors. Bob was a heavy smoker for a number of years and found that in his seventies he'd lost much of his ability to taste and smell, which inhibited his enjoyment of eating and sharing a meal with others.[6]

What can you do? Try new foods, such as ethnic foods, that use a variety of herbs and spices, which will stimulate your sense of taste and smell. Change your menu to add variety and new tastes and smells. Try aromatherapy and enjoy a wide range of smells.

Touch: When you touch something your brain interprets the type and amount of sensation. It also interprets the sensation as pleasant or unpleasant. Many studies have shown that with aging, you may have reduced or changed sensations of pain, vibration, cold, heat, pressure, and touch. It may be that some of the normal changes of aging are caused by decreased blood flow to the touch receptors or to the brain and spinal cord. The increasing inability to discern between temperatures, vibration, touch, and pressure, and decreased sensitivity to pain can increase risk of injuries. Darlene was surprised to find she'd burned herself after touching a shelf in her oven that didn't feel as hot as it actually was.[7]

What can you do? Dig in your garden with your hands, try a pottery class, make cookies and mix the dough with your hands, gently caress your spouse's neck (or add massage to your intimate times together), stroke your cat until it purrs, try to catch your goldfish without looking into the bowl—

any activity that keeps those touch receptors and your brain alive and well.

Proprioception: This is often referred to as our sixth sense and is critically important to our everyday function even though it is so unconscious that few even know it is there. "Proprioception refers to the brain's ability to know where our body is in space. The brain gathers information from a wide range of senses and then processes this information in order to compare it with a virtual body map . . . stored in our memory."[8] Without this important sense we might walk into door frames, bump into people as we pass them on the sidewalk or in a crowded room, and not be able to judge how close we are coming to the curb as we drive. This sense allows us to generate and maintain our upright posture and physical balance. If our body-in-space sense is diminished we must tune up all our other senses to compensate, which can lead to tiredness or loss of concentration.

Many Baby Boomers have experienced deterioration in these important areas and are dismayed as they glance at themselves in the mirror, shocked at their slumping posture. Or they're surprised to have difficulty riding a bicycle or ice skating, which they used to do with ease. To maintain balance, our sixth sense works closely with the vestibular system of the inner ear.

As we age it is important to strengthen and maintain our sixth sense, and this is often accomplished by putting time and energy into balance and core training. Core training integrates the abdominal, gluteal, lumbar, and groin muscles and tissues. This is one way to help keep our sixth sense in good working order.

What can you do? Activities that challenge your balance like balancing on a wobble board in the gym or taking a Pilates class. Practice standing on one leg while lifting light weights for a good workout. Muscles do have a memory, and even though it may have been years since you engaged a particular group of muscles they will still "fire" and with time may enable you not only to unconsciously stand tall and walk like a young adult, but also improve your badminton, bocce, bowling, croquet, horseshoes, shuffleboard, and maybe even your golf game.

| 39 |

Understand How Alcohol Affects Your Brain

If you drink, don't drive, don't even putt.

—Dean Martin[1]

One way to understand how our brain is affected by alcohol is to follow the path of a glass of wine. With the first sip, alcohol floods the GI tract, is absorbed by the small intestine, forges into the liver for filtration, and empties into the blood stream, flowing to the heart and the brain. Once in the brain, alcohol affects a number of major areas including the frontal lobes (learning and memory) and the cerebellum (movement and coordination).

According to the National Council on Alcohol and Drug Dependence (NCADD), "Alcohol is metabolized extremely quickly by the body. Unlike foods, which require time for digestion, alcohol needs no digestion and is quickly absorbed.

Alcohol gets 'VIP' treatment in the body, absorbing and metabolizing before most other nutrients. About 20 percent is absorbed directly across the walls of an empty stomach and can reach the brain within one minute.

"Alcohol is rapidly absorbed in the upper portion of the small intestine. The alcohol-laden blood then travels to the liver via the veins and capillaries of the digestive tract, which affects nearly every liver cell. The liver cells are the only cells in our body that can produce enough of the enzyme alcohol dehydrogenase to oxidize alcohol at an appreciable rate.

"Though alcohol affects every organ of the body, its most dramatic impact is upon the liver. . . . when alcohol is present, the liver cells are forced to first metabolize the alcohol, letting the fatty acids accumulate, sometimes in huge amounts. Alcohol metabolism permanently changes liver cell structure, which impairs the liver's ability to metabolize fats. . . .

"The liver is able to metabolize about ½ ounce of ethanol per hour (approximately one drink, depending on a person's body size, food intake, etc.). If more alcohol arrives in the liver than the enzymes can handle, the excess alcohol travels to all parts of the body, circulating until the liver enzymes are finally able to process it."[2]

Alcohol's effect on the brain is a good news-bad news scenario. First the good news. Drinking moderate amounts of alcohol appears to reduce the risk of dementia and Alzheimer's disease. "Researchers studied individuals participating in the Rotterdam Study (7,983 people aged 55 or older) over an average period of six years. Those who consumed one to three drinks of alcohol per day had a significantly lower risk of dementia (including Alzheimer's) than did abstainers."[3]

On the down side, most are very familiar with the dangerous effect of long-term heavy drinking upon the liver and brain. We know that drinking alcohol clearly affects the brain as we observe "party-goers" becoming relaxed and happy and maybe even a little unsteady. That quiet chap transforms into the life of the party after just a couple beers. This effect may seem so mild and transient that few give thought to the fact that alcohol could turn sinister and *permanently* affect the brain in negative ways with frequent or heavy drinking. A host of factors influence this possibility including: how much alcohol is consumed, age, gender, how long a person has been drinking, genetics, and general health. All too many college students engage in "binge drinking," defined as consuming five or more drinks in two hours for men and four or more for women. This practice has been blamed for many serious health problems and even deaths on college campuses.

Researchers are continuing to study short- and long-term effects of alcohol upon the brain, using modern technology such as MRI and PET imaging to pinpoint damage. "These snapshots of the living brain show disturbances in the way brain cells communicate as well as on blood flow and metabolism in the brain. . . . Studies have proven that long-term heavy drinking may lead to shrinking of the brain as well as deficiencies in the white matter that carries information between brain cells. Damage in the brains of alcoholics is shown in regions associated with learning and memory as well as the cerebellum which controls movement and coordination."[4]

As many as 80 percent of those addicted to alcohol are deficient in the vitamin thiamin. This deficiency alone can lead to twenty-five serious conditions, which together are named Wernicke-Korsakoff's Syndrome. Even the milder version may include confusion, muscle uncoordination, and a temporary paralysis of the nerves involved in eye movements.[5]

Many of these changes are reversible with abstinence and the help of various medications. The explosion of research and new knowledge about how our brain can regenerate has brought hope for reversing alcohol-related brain damage, but prevention is always superior to trying to undo damage that has occurred.

The bottom line is that it is up to *you* to become aware of alcohol's influence on *you*, and to learn to handle it responsibly. Perhaps more than any other health-related practice, alcohol use is an area where we can be our brain's best friend or worst enemy, with no one to blame but ourselves, as the famous Jimmy Buffett song "Margaritaville" admits.

The first step is to understand how alcohol affects our own individual brain. We are so uniquely created that there is never going to be a "safe list" of alcohol-related behaviors that will apply to all people. To drink *responsibly* we need to learn our own individual limits and conscientiously avoid crossing the line into alcohol abuse. Even this, however, can be one of those "best laid plans" that often go astray, as a person slips gradually into dependence on this substance to feel "normal" (or to dull the pain) only to find that there's a really good reason for the term "demon rum"; specifically, that alcohol (especially hard liquor) can seem to possess such strong powers that casting it out or casting it away takes everything you've got. And then, it just takes one drink to renew those strong synaptic connections lurking in the central amygdala of your brain, just waiting for some more of that concoction (again in Buffett's words) that helps you hang on.

If you know exactly what we mean here because you've experienced it, or are experiencing it, please seek help from a qualified medical professional. If you don't understand what this paragraph means, be glad . . . but also be gracious to those who are in or have been in alcohol's grip. If you drink daily, wonder how it is affecting you, but aren't concerned enough to quit, honestly answer these questions (posted on the NCADD site):

- Do you have a problem with alcohol?
- Have you ever felt you should cut down on your drinking?
- Are you annoyed when people criticize your drinking?
- Have you ever felt bad or guilty about your drinking?
- Have you ever had a drink the first thing in the morning to steady your nerves or get rid of a hangover?

If you answered "yes" to one question, you may have a problem with alcohol. More than one "yes" answer makes it highly likely that a problem exists. "Yes" to all of them could be the first draft of your epitaph, should you continue to pretend that the statistics always apply to somebody else.

| 40 |

Worship God in Spirit and Truth*

God is spirit, and his worshipers must worship in spirit and
in truth.

—Jesus (John 4:24 NIV)

Everyone worships something. And what we choose to worship has a deep effect on our health, including the health of
our minds. For is it not rational to say this: worship something
that cannot save you, you are deceived; worship something
that can save you, you are wise.

According to psychiatrist Timothy R. Jennings, MD, the
drive to worship is "an inherent part of our being . . . experienced by everyone, whether they admit it or not. It might be
the Dallas Cowboys, money, power, a pop culture figure such

---

*Please note that this chapter is more specifically focused on the importance of
religion to brain health than any other in this book. We trust you will read it with
an open mind.

as Madonna, the scientific method, or oneself. But everyone worships something."[1] To this list we might add a variety of other things that people worship, including sex, fame, one's spouse or family, external beauty, automobiles, NASCAR cars and drivers, Indy cars and drivers, yachts, houses and properties, technologies, politicians and their ideologies, religious leaders and their ideologies, Hollywood personalities, TV, heroes (athletic and otherwise), rock music, classical music, psychedelic experiences, physical fitness, health, longevity, relics, saints, ancestors, hunting, fishing, surfing, rats, golden calves and sacred cows, even shoes . . . the list of things people are willing to consider sacred is as long as the number of people in the world is large. An article I (Dave) received while creating this chapter included a conversation between the missionary doctor and the patient, who responded to the question, "What do you worship?" by pulling a little jade Buddha from her pocket. "This is what I worship," she replied.

In Athens, in the apostle Paul's day, there was an altar in the Areopagus to "an unknown god."[2] And the apostle used that innate belief—that there was something greater—to speak of Jesus and the gospel. This is exactly what took place, word for word, from Acts 17:22–32 (NIV):

Paul then stood up in the meeting of the Areopagus and said: "Men of Athens! I see that in every way you are very religious. For as I walked around and looked carefully at your objects of worship, I even found an altar with this inscription: To AN UNKNOWN GOD. Now what you worship as something unknown I am going to proclaim to you. The God who made the world and everything in it is the Lord of heaven and earth and does not live in temples built by hands. And he is not served by human hands, as if he needed anything, because he himself gives all men life and breath and everything else.

From one man he made every nation of men, that they should inhabit the whole earth; and he determined the times set for them and the exact places where they should live. God did this so that men would seek him and perhaps reach out for him and find him, though he is not far from each one of us. 'For in him we live and move and have our being.' As some of your own poets have said, 'We are his offspring.' Therefore since we are God's offspring, we should not think that the divine being is like gold or silver or stone—an image made by man's design and skill. In the past God overlooked such ignorance, but now he commands all people everywhere to repent. For he has set a day when he will judge the world with justice by the man he has appointed. He has given proof of this to all men by raising him from the dead." When they heard about the resurrection of the dead, some of them sneered, but others said, "We want to hear you again on this subject."

Fast forward nearly 2,000 years: Freud, the "father" of modern psychotherapy, describes religion as a form of neurosis, and Marx, the father of communism, calls religion the opiate of the people (this was before the 1960s turned opiates into the religion of the people). Their opinions and writings could not bury the truth that all human beings are religious to one degree or another, if by "religious" we mean that they exhibit a certain level of faithful devotion to an ultimate reality or deity. The Judeo-Christian tradition is clear on the reason for this, since both Old and New Testaments describe this innate human need to worship and the consequences of worshiping truth versus a lie.

For example, the Old Testament prophet Isaiah wrote: "Half of the wood he burns in the fire . . . From the rest he makes a god, his idol; he bows down to it and worships. He prays to it and says, 'Save me; you are my god.' They know nothing, they understand nothing; their eyes are plastered over so they cannot see, and their minds closed so they cannot understand. No one stops to think, no one has the knowledge or understanding to say, 'Half of it I used for fuel; I even baked bread over its coals, I roasted meat and I ate. Shall I make a detestable thing from what is left? Shall I bow down to a block of wood?' He feeds on ashes, a deluded heart misleads him; he cannot save himself, or say, 'Is not this thing in my right hand a lie?' " (Isa. 44:16–20, NIV).

The New Testament is equally clear: "For since the creation of the world God's invisible qualities—his eternal power and divine nature—have been clearly seen, being understood from what has been made, so that men are without excuse. For although they knew God, they neither glorified him as God nor gave thanks to him, but their thinking became futile and their foolish hearts were darkened. Although they claimed to be wise, they became fools and exchanged the glory of the immortal God for images made to look like mortal man and birds and animals and reptiles. . . . They exchanged the truth of God for a lie, and worshiped and served created things rather than the Creator—who is forever praised. Amen. . . . Furthermore, since they did not think it worthwhile to retain the knowledge of God, he gave them over to a depraved mind. . . ." (Rom. 1:20–28, NIV).

Since all humans in all ages have worshiped something, there is obviously an innate drive in this direction. If you accept the idea of a Creator God, then it is clear, and fairly painlessly so, that the Creator made us this way. If you do not accept the concept of a Creator, or Intelligent Design, or whatever you wish to call it, then you simply cannot explain this drive, whether you appeal to Freud, Marx, Darwin, or anybody else.

Lest we seem to be claiming some superiority of knowledge or faith, we want you to know that even when we believe in such a Creator God—whom we seek to worship in spirit and truth—we can still get so caught up in our temporal viewpoint about the way things are or ought to be that we lose sight of the eternal, which is where He dwells. When this happens, we may "lose our minds" for awhile, until we anchor them again to the solid rock.

I (Dave) could tell you many stories of how this has happened for me, most of them contained in my earlier books: *Jonathan, You Left Too Soon* and *If God Is So Good, Why Do I Hurt So Bad?* But to illustrate this point—that even when we have faith, it is still subject to human emotions and other factors that can render us temporarily "insane"—let me share a short story regarding something that happened after the death of my first son, when I held myself responsible and was unable to force my reason to control my emotions, with the result that I was simply and unambiguously guilty, guilty, guilty.

To avoid adding to my weight of guilt, I tried to do everything right. It didn't matter that this goal was impossible, in practice. What mattered most (to my sick mind) was that any intentional or unintentional failure just pressed me down further (which is a very good definition of depression, by the way). Once when I was driving along (I was the pastor of a small church in the Upper Peninsula of Michigan at the time) I saw what seemed to be an inordinate amount of smoke coming from the chimney of a home I passed. I drove on a bit, then turned around and drove back to check that the home was not on fire. Then, I had to do it one more time, to be absolutely sure that I hadn't missed something that might help a family avoid dying tragically in a fire. What I didn't realize at the time was that, as magnanimous as this motive may sound, I was in reality trying to save myself from adding more guilt to an already overwhelmingly heavy load.[3]

The only way out of such a mind trap is to remember who God really is, and to accept His grace and forgiveness, since as Jesus said, "The truth will set you free" (John 8:32, NIV), the corollary being that the "lie" will never set you free. This applies to believers and nonbelievers, too. We really mean it when we say that you're welcome to believe what you want to believe. But if you want peace of mind, and health of mind, you'll survey all of history and all of religion, philosophy, and psychology, and any other discipline, and you'll see that in the end there was one person who was unique. He lived to show us what God is like. He died to take away our sins, so we might have life more abundantly, and He rose again from the dead to defeat our ultimate adversary, death, of which all our weaknesses and all our failures, including our attempts to keep our minds, not lose them, are but poor reflections of what is to come, without Him. But then again, with Him, all is well and will be well, with body, soul, and mind.

Notes

Introduction

1. William P. Cheshire Jr., MD, "Grey Matters: In the Twilight of Aging, a Twinkle of Hope," *Ethics & Medicine* 24, no. 1 (Spring 2008): 9.

2. Zach Lynch, *The Neuro Revolution: How Brain Science is Changing Our World* (New York: St. Martin's Press, 2009), 10.

3. Ibid., 4.

4. Alvaro Fernandez and Dr. Elkhonon Goldberg, *The SharpBrains Guide to Brain Fitness* (San Francisco: SharpBrains, Inc., 2009), xiv.

5. Ibid., 8.

Chapter 1 Alter Your Brain with Prayer and Meditation

1. Daniel Amen, "Healing the Hardware of the Soul," *Christian Counseling Today* 12, no. 3 (2004): 19–24.

2. Ibid.

3. Andrew Newberg and Mark Robert Waldman, *How God Changes Your Brain* (New York: Ballantine Books, 2009), 18–19.

4. Ibid., 27.

5. Andrew Newberg, M. Pourdehnad, et al, "Cerebral blood flow during meditative prayer: preliminary findings and methodological issues," *Perceptual & Motor Skills* 97, no. 2 (2003): 625–30.

Chapter 2 Ask: Is It Alzheimer's, Aging, or Stress?

1. Quoted by the European College of Neuropsychopharmacology, 22 Congress, September 12–16, 2009.

2. N. R. Kleinfield, "More than Death, Fearing a Muddled Mind," *The New York Times*, November 11, 2002, http://www.nytimes.com/2002/11/11/nyrefion/more-than-death-fearing-a-muddled-mind.html.

3. "Oleocanthal may help prevent, treat Alzheimer's," Monell Chemical Senses Center, September 29, 2009, http://www.monell.org.

4. "Saturated Fats Can Cause Alzheimer's Disease," Health and Finance Update: Latest News and Reviews, http://news-reviews.org/uncategorized/saturated-fats-can-cuase-alzheimers-disease/.

5. Jean Carper, *Your Miracle Brain* (New York: Harper Collins, 2000), 23.

6. Ibid.

7. Daniel J. DeNoon, "Mediterranean Diet Plus Exercise Lowers Alzheimer's Risk," http://www.webmd.com/alzheimers/news/20090811/mediterranean-diet-plus-exercise-cuts-alzheimers-risk?page=1.

8. "Early warning signs of Alzheimer's updated for earlier detection," Alzheimer's Association, *Kako'o: The Aloha Chapter Newsletter* (27: 2, Summer 2009).

Chapter 3 Avoid Dirty Water

1. "Water, sanitation and hygiene links to health," World Health Organization, http://who.int/water_sanitation_health/publications/facts2004/en/print.html.

2. http://www.epa.gov/safewater/lead/pdfs.

3. Kathleen Doheny, "Bacteria May Lurk on Your Showerhead," http://www.webmd.com/lung/copd/news/20090914/bacteria-may-lurk-on-your-showerhead.

4. "Water Treatment Methods," Centers for Disease Control and Prevention, http://wwwnc.cdc.gov/travel/content/water-treatment.aspx.

5. "Lead in Paint, Dust, and Soil," U.S. EPA, http://www.epa.gov/lead/pubs/leadinfo.htm.

6. See the section on the pork tapeworm, in the chapter "Don't Eat Squirrel Brains." Other potential dangers to the brain from drinking untreated mountain water might involve ingesting contaminants from wild animals with central nervous system diseases.

7. "Healthy Swimming/Recreational Water," Centers for Disease Control and Prevention, http://www.cdc.gov/healthywater/swimming/index.html.

Chapter 4 Become a Lifelong Learner

1. Michael Merzenich, "Engage Your Brain," AARP, http://www.aarp.org/health/brain/takingcontrol/engage_your_brain.html.

2. Denise C. Park, Angela H. Gutchess, Michelle L. Meade, and Elizabeth A. L. Stine-Morrow, "Improving Cognitive Function in Older Adults: Nontraditional Approaches," *Journals of Gerontology*: SERIES B 62B (Special Issue I, 2007): 45–52.

3. K. M. Lang, D. Llewellyn, I. Lang, D. Weir, R. Wallace, M. Kabeto, and F. Huppert, "Cognitive Health Among Older Adults In The United States and in England," *BMC Geriatrics* (2009, 9): 23.

4. Lewis Lajos Incze. *Footprints on Destiny Lane* (Lisbon Falls, ME: Beacon Press), 1982.

5. S. L. Willis, et al, "Long-term Effects of Cognitive Training on Everyday Functional Outcomes in Older Adults," *Journal of American Medical Association* (296:23): 2805–14.

Chapter 5 Brain Safe Your Home

1. "Clinical Guidance for Carbon Monoxide (CO) Poisoning After a Disaster," Centers for Disease Control and Prevention, http://emergency.cdc.gov/disasters/co_guidance.asp.

2. "Lead," Centers for Disease Control and Prevention, http://www.cdc.gov/nceh/lead/.

3. For more information on this, see the book *Finding Your Way After the Suicide of Someone You Love*, by David B. Biebel and Suzanne Foster (Grand Rapids: Zondervan, 2005).

4. "Teenager Dies After Inhaling Dust-Off Cleaning Spray," http://urbanlegends.about.com/library/bl_dust_off.htm.

Chapter 6 Discover Something

1. Carper, *Your Miracle Brain*, 2.

2. Charles Q. Choi, "Eureka! Brain's discovery circuits found," http://www.msnbc.msn.com/id/22806180/.

3. "University of Pittsburgh led study maps the making of a decision in the human brain," *Virtual Medical Worlds*, October 2007, http://www.hoise.com/vmw/07/articles/vmw/LV-VM-11-07-33.html.

4. http://www.melfisher.com/.

5. "Inspirational Quotes To Keep You Inspired and Motivated," http://www.great-inspirational-quotes.com/inspirational-quotes.html.

Chapter 7 Discover Your Gold Mind

1. Carper, *Your Miracle Brain*, 5–7.

2. "MIT: Brain's Messengers Could Be Regulated-Potential for Better Understanding of Schizophrenia," *Medical News Today*, September 17, 2007, http://www.medicalnewstoday.com/printerfriendlynews.php?newsid=82530.

3. David B. Biebel, and Harold G. Koenig, *New Light On Depression* (Grand Rapids: Zondervan, 2004), 171–72, used by permission of the book authors and Forrest, the author of the self-report.

4. For information related to nutrition and brain health, contact us at: DBBV1@aol.com.

Chapter 8 Dodge a Stroke

1. John Gullotta, "Taking Stock for Stroke Prevention, Australian Medical Association," Medical News Today, September 2008, www.medicalnewstoday.com/printerfriendlynews.php?newsid=121601.

2. "Stroke Facts and Statistics," CDC, http://www.cdc.gov/stroke/stroke_facts.htm.

3. Ibid.

4. Diana Rodriguez, "The 'Stroke Belt': Why Is Stroke Risk Higher in the Southeast?" http://www.everydayhealth.com/stroke/stroke-risk-higher-in-southeastern-us.aspx.

5. "Stroke Prevention," CDC, http://www.cdc.gov/stroke/prevention.htm.

6. "Cholesterol Control Plus Blood Pressure Control Equals Stroke Prevention," Medical News Today, April 2009, www.medicalnewstoday.com/printerfriendlynews.php?newsid=148273.

Chapter 9 Don't Eat Squirrel Brains

1. Charles Wolfe, "Squirrel Brains May Be Unsafe," http://www.greysquirrel.net/brain.html.

2. Sandra Blakeslee, "Kentucky Doctors Warn Against a Regional Dish: Squirrels' Brains," *The New York Times*, August 29, 1997, http://www.nytimes.com/1997/08/29/us/kentucky-doctors-warn-against-a-regional-dish-squirrels-brains.html.

3. Findings were published in *The Lancet* (350, no. 9078: August 30, 1997), http://www.mad-cow.org/~tom/victim23.html.

4. Wolfe, "Squirrel Brains."

5. "Bovine spongiform encephalopathy," Wikipedia, http://en.wikipedia.org/wiki/Bovine_spongiform_encephalopathy.

6. "Cow Brain Sandwiches Still on the Menu," http://www.rense.com/general47/still.htm.

7. "Prion," Wikipedia, http://en.wikipedia.org/wiki/Prion#cite_note-ictvdb-prions-29.

8. Lauren Cox, "It's Not a Tumor, It's a Brain Worm," ABC News, http://abcnews.go.com/Health/PainManagement/story?id=6309464&page=1&page=1.

9. Andrew Banyai, "The Lure of Discovery, Thrill of Danger and Hidden Hazards of Arctic Exploration," *Chest* (vol. 59, no. 1, January 1971), http://chestjournal.chestpubs.org/content/59/1/46.full.pdf.

Chapter 10 Don't Let Your Habits Become Addictions

1. "Addiction Quotes," Great-Quotes.com, http://www.great-quotes.com/quotes/category/Addiction.htm.

2. Michael Lemonick, "How We Get Addicted," *Time*, July 5, 2007, http://www.time.com/time/magazine/article/0,9171,1640436,00.html.

3. Ruth Engs, adapted from *Alcohol and Other Drugs: Self Responsibility* (Bloomington, IN: Tichenor Publishing Company, 1987), http://www.indiana.edu/~engs/hints/addictiveb.html.http://www.indiana.edu/~engs/rbook/readabd.htm.

4. "Addiction and Brain Activity: What Happens in the Brain," *Time*, 2007, http://www.time.com/time/2007/addiction/.

5. Lemonick, "How We Get Addicted."

6. Engs, *Alcohol and Other Drugs*.

7. Ibid.

8. Ibid.

9. Marnie C. Ferree, *No Stones* (Xulon Press, 2002).

10. *Jakarta Globe*, "Pornography Addiction May Cause Brain Damage in Kids?" (2009), http://addictionsawareness.com/2009/03/pornography-addiction-may-cause-brain-damage-in-kids/.

11. Heather Hatfield, "Shopping Spree, or Addiction?" WebMD, 2004, http://www.webmd.com/mental-health/features/shopping-spree-addiction.

12. Engs, *Alcohol and Other Drugs*.

Chapter 11 Eat Safe Fish

1. "Frequently Asked Questions About PCBs Found in Trout," http://www.fish.state.pa.us/qpcb2001.htm.
2. A copy of the report is posted at: http://water.usgs.gov/nawqa/mercury/.
3. "What You Need to Know About Mercury in Fish and Shellfish," (US EPA: EPA-823-F-04-009).
4. "Is Fish Really Brain Food?" http://www.wellnessletter.com/html/wl/2001/wlFeatured1001.html.

Chapter 12 Embrace the Digital Age

1. "History of the internet," Wikipedia, http://en.wikipedia.org/wiki/History_of_the_internet.
2. "UCLA study finds that searching the internet increases brain function," Physorg.com, http://www.physorg.com/news143205108.html.

Chapter 13 Enjoy Sports

1. "Sports Quotes," Thinkexist.com,http://thinkexist.com/quotations/sports/2.html.
2. Vogt, Heidi, "Meet the Women who Watch Sports," *Media Life Magazine*, November 15, 2002, http://www.medialifemagazine.com/news2002/nov02/nov11/5_fri/news1friday.html.
3. "Professional Football Still America's Favorite Sport," The Harris Poll, 2008, http://www.harrisinteractive.com/harris_poll/index.asp?PID=866.
4. "How Walking Buffs Your Brain," AARP, June 2004, http://www.aarp.org/health/brain-health/info-2004/walking_brain_booster.html.
5. "Playing, and Even Watching, Sports Improves Brain Function," *Science Daily*, September 3, 2008, http://www.sciencedaily.com/releases/2008/09/080901205631.htm.
6. Ibid.
7. Ibid.

Chapter 14 Equip Your Brain by Exercising Your Heart

1. "Heart health and lifestyle help seniors maintain brain power," February 22, 2006, http://www.news-medical.net/news/2006/02/22/16130.aspx.
2. Bradley Hatfield, University of Maryland, College Park, School of Public Health, "Exercise Benefits Aging Brain, Alzheimer's," October 26, 2007, http://www.newsdesk.umd.edu/scitech/release.cfm?ArticleID=1532.

3. "Exercise in moderation best for the brain," *Medical Research News*, November 28, 2005, www.news-medical.net/print_article.asp?id= 14724.

4. "Exercise gives the brain a workout, too," CBS Evening News, January 30, 2009, www.cbsnews.com/stories/2009/01/30/earlyshow/health/main4764523.shtml.

Chapter 15 Feed Your Neurons Well

1. "Coffee is number one source of antioxidants," Physorg.com, http://www.physorg.com/news6067.html.

2. Hannes B. Staehelin, "Micronutrients and Alzheimer's disease," Proceedings of the Nutrition Society (2005, 64): 565-570.

3. Contact us (see back pages) for information on how to accomplish this.

4. "Higher Cognitive Performance with High Intake of Fruits and Vegetables," Elements4Health.com, http://www.elements4health.com/higher-cognitive-performance-with-high-intake-of-fruits-and-vegetables.html.

5. "Free radical theory of aging," Wikipedia, http://en.wikipedia.org/wiki/Free_radical_theory_of_aging.

6. Marlo Sollitto, "Power Foods: Doctors' Top Choices for Antioxidant Rich Foods," http://www.agingcare.com/Featured-Stories/113293/Power-Foods-Doctors-Top-Choices-for-Antioxidant-Rich-Foods.htm.

7. "What's good for your heart is good for your brain," Alz.org, http://www.alz.org/heartbrain/overviewh2.asp.

8. For information on this option, contact us.

Chapter 16 Get Off the Couch

1. "Couch potato," Answers.com, http://www.answers.com/topic/couch-potato.

2. Ibid.

3. Doc Gurley, "Is Your Brain a Couch Potato?" Sfgate.com, June 8, 2009, http://www.sfgate.com/cgi-bin/blogs/gurley/detail?entry_id=41335#ixzz0XXBeoiE3.

4. MindSparke, http://www.mindsparke.com/?gclid=CP7y9KeGrp4CFc5L5Qod8jQzpA.

5. The following is excerpted from a letter posted by the developer of MindSparke in response to an article on the subject of neurogenesis by Matt

Perry (http://www.newsreview.com/sacramento/content?oid=1263769):
Posted 09/24/2009 11:32AM by MindSparke

Hello, Matt. Thank you for giving such a comprehensive overview of the state of the brain fitness arena. I would like to point out that critics of brain training such as Dr. Knopman may mislead people into thinking that there is no reliable and impressive academic evidence of what brain training programs can do. Quite the contrary, brain training can achieve results that far surpass anything possible with normal engagement in everyday life. A joint Michigan and Bern University study last year "Improving Fluid Intelligence by Training Working Memory (PNAS April 2008)" recorded increases in mental agility (fluid intelligence) of more than 40% after 19 days of focused brain training. This kind of trained improvement is remarkable and demonstrates just how effective the right brain training can be. We use the same protocol in our software (Mind Sparke Brain Fitness Pro), which is one of the programs available at the vibrantBrains facilities, as well as online. Martin Walker www.mindsparke.com Effective, Affordable Brain Training Software.

6. Alvaro Fernandez and Dr. Elkhonon Goldberg, *The SharpBrains Guide to Brain Fitness* (San Francisco: SharpBrains, Inc., 2009), 8–9.

Chapter 17 Go to Church

1. From verse 2 of the hymn "Tell Me the Old, Old Story," lyrics by A. Katherine Hankey, 1866.

2. Terrence D. Hill, "Religion, Spirituality, and Healthy Cognitive Aging," *Southern Medical Journal* (99, no. 10, 2006): 1176–77.

3. Ibid.

4. "Reading 'can help reduce stress'," telegraph.co.uk, March 30, 2009, http://www.telegraph.co.uk/health/healthnews/5070874/Reading-can-help-reduce-stress.html.

Chapter 18 Improve Your Thinking Day by Day

1. Simon Wootton and Terry Horne, "The Heirarchy of Thinking Skills," *Training Your Brain* (Blacklick, OH: McGraw Hill Co., 2007), 61.

2. *ESRC Society Today.* "Children are falling behind in math and science." http://www.esrc.ac.uk/ESRCInfoCentre/about/CI/CP/the_edge/issue21/maths_science.aspx.

3. Alvaro Fernandez, "ABC Reporter Bob Woodruff's Incredible Recovery from Traumatic Brain Injury," September 15, 2008, http://www.huffingtonpost.com/alvaro-fernandez/abc-reporter-bob-woodruff_b_125863.html.

Chapter 19 Keep Your Nose Clean

1. Diane Ackerman, *A Natural History of the Senses* (New York: Vintage Books, 1990), xv.

2. Ibid., 5.

3. "Loss of Smell Linked to Key Protein in Alzheimer's Disease," *Science Daily*, March 12, 2004, http://www.sciencedaily.com/releases/2004/03/040312090410.htm.

4. Ibid.

5. "Decrease in Sense of Smell Seen in Lupus Patients," *Science Daily*, May 6, 2009, http://www.sciencedaily.com/releases/2009/04/090430161230.htm.

6. Study published by the University of Maryland Medical Center, "Parkinson's disease—Diagnosis," http://www.umm.edu/parkinsons/diagnosis.htm.

7. "Danger triangle of the face," Wikipedia, http://en.wikipedia.org/wiki/Danger_triangle_of_the_face.

Chapter 20 Know How Your Meds Affect Your Brain

1. Campbell Noll, Malaz Boustani, Tony Limbil, et al, "Commonly Used Medications May Produce Cognitive Impairment in Seniors," *Journal of Clinical Interventions in Aging* (June 5, 2009).

2. "Seniors & Drugs Prescription Peril Eases With Beers List," CBC News, September 13, 2007, http://www.cbc.ca/news/background/seniorsdrugs/.

3. Rita Carter, et al, *The Human Brain Book* (London, New York, Melbourne, Munich, and Delhi: DK Adult, 2009), 128.

4. Marc Ramirez, "More Die From Drugs Than Traffic Accidents," *The Seattle Times*, October 2, 2009, http://seattletimes.nwsource.com/cgi-bin/PrintStory.pl?document_id=2009985051&zsection.

5. Ibid.

Chapter 21 Learn a New Language

1. J. W. King and Richard Suzman, "Prospects for Improving Cognition Throughout the Life Course," *Psychological Science in the Public Interest*, (vol. 9, no. 1, 2003): ii.

2. T. Kanaya, M. H. Scullin, and S. J. Ceci, "The Flynn Effect and U.S. Policies," *American Psychologist* (vol. 58, no. 10): 778–90.

3. Melonie Heron, et al, "Deaths: Final Data for 2006," *National Vital Statistics Reports* (57, no. 14, 2009).

4. S. Ge, C. Yang, K. Hsu, G. Ming, and H. Song, "A Critical Period of Enhanced Synaptic Plasticity In Newly Generated Neurons of the Adult Brain," *Neuron* (54, 2007): 559–66.

Chapter 22 Learn to Paint

1. William H. Calvin, *The Throwing Madonna: Essays on the Brain* (New York: Bantam, 1991).

2. M. S. Gazzaniga, "Cerebral specialization and interhemispheric communication, Does the corpus callosum enable the human condition?" *Brain* (123: 7, 2000): 1293–1326.

3. Iain McGilchrist, "The Battle Between the Brain's Right and Left Hemispheres," adapted from his book, *The Master and his Emissary: the Divided Brain and the Making of the Western World* (New Haven: Yale University Press, 2009), http://current.com/items/91885213_the-battle-between-the-brains-left-and-right-hemispheres.htm.

4. T. M. Chamberlin Hodgson, B. Parris, M. James, N. Gutowski, M. Hussain, and C. Kennard, "The role of the ventral frontal cortex in inhibitory oculomotor control," *Brain* (130: 6, 2007): 1525–37.

5. Henry Ward Beecher, *Proverbs from Plymouth Pulpit*, 1887.

Chapter 23 Memorize

1. See: Thinkexist.com, www.thinkexist.com/English/topic/x/topic_271_3.html.

2. "Scientists Show Hippocampus's Role in Long Term Memory," *Science Daily*, 2004, www.sciencedaily.com/releases/2004/05/040513010413.htm.

3. Simon Wootton and Terry Horne, *Training Your Brain* (Blacklick, OH: McGraw-Hill Companies, Inc., 2007), 79.

4. "Researchers Show How The Hippocampus Records Memory," http://www.news-medical.net/news/2009/03/12/46843.ASPX.

Chapter 24 Mind Your Head

1. Hana Lee, Max Wintermark, et al, "Focal Lesions in Acute Mile Traumatic Brain Injury and Neurocognitive Outcome: CT versus 3T MRI," *Journal of Neurotrauma* (September 25, 2008): 1049.

2. "Concussion," American Association of Neurological Surgeons, http://www.neurosurgerytoday.org/what/patient_e/concussion.asp.
3. "Study Links Concussions to Brain Disease," CBS News, http://www.cbsnews.com/stories/2009/10/09/60minutes/main5371686.shtml?t ag=contentMain;cbsCarousel.
4. Ibid.
5. "Concussion and Mild TBI," CDC, http://www.cdc.gov/concussion/.
6. "The Top 5 Causes of Head Injuries and How to Avoid Them," SixWise.com, http://www.sixwise.com/newsletters/05/09/28/the-top-5-causes-of-head-injuries-and-how-to-avoid-them.htm.
7. Ibid.
8. http://www.braintrauma.org/site/PageServer?pagename=TBI_Facts.
9. See http://www.cdc.gov/TraumaticBrainInjury/tbi_concussion.html.

Chapter 25 Pay Attention to the Brain in Your Gut

1. See Thinkexist.com, http://www.thinkExist.com/quotes/with/keyword/gut.
2. "The Brain Gut Axis," http://www.ibsresearchupdate.org/IBS/brain1ie4.html.
3. Douglas Drossman, et al, "A Focus Group Assessment of Patients' Perspectives on Irritable Bowel Syndrome and Illness Severity," *Digestive Disease Science* (54: 7, July 2009): 1532–41.

Chapter 26 Play Mind-Friendly Games

1. See Thinkexist.com, http://thinkexist.com/quotes/with/keyword/game/2.html.
2. "Want to Improve Memory? Strengthen Your Synapses. Here's How," *Medical News Today* (January 2007), http://www.medicalnewstoday.com/articles/60455.php.
3. Ibid.
4. Steven Johnson, "Your Brain on Video Games," *Discover Magazine*, July, 2005, http://discovermagazine.com/2005/jul/brain-on-video-games.

Chapter 27 Practice Positive Self-Talk

1. "Self-Talk," Great-Quotes.com, http://www.great-quotes.com/quotes/category/Self-Talk.htm.

2. Ibid.

3. Dorothy Neddermeyer, Ph.D, "Positive Self-Talk to Achieve Goals," Ezine Articles, 2006, http://ezinearticles.com/?Positive-Self-Talk-to-Achieve-Goals&id=397941.

4. Ibid.

5. From Philippians 4: "We've Got Mail," a paraphrase of the New Testament epistles by Rev. Warren C. Biebel, *We've Got Mail* (Roseland, FL: Healthy Life Press, 2009), 58.

Chapter 28 Protect Your Brain from Insects

1. P. D. Baz, *A Dictionary of Proverbs* (New York: Philosophical Library, Inc., 1963), 169.

2. CDC Lyme Disease Homepage, http://www.wrongdiagnosis.com/artic/cdc_lyme_disease_home_page_dvbid.htm.

3. "West Nile virus," Wikipedia, http://en.wikipedia.org/wiki/West_Nile_virus.

4. "West Nile Virus: What You Need To Know," CDC, http://www.cdc.gov/ncidod/dvbid/westnile/wnv_factsheet.htm.

5. "Updated Information Regarding Insect Repellents," CDC, http://www.cdc.gov/ncidod/dvbid/westnile/RepellentUpdates.htm.

6. "Insect Repellent: Best Insect Repellent for Kids," http://pediatrics.about.com/od/childhoodmedications/a/609_insect_repl.htm.

7. "Insect repellents: which keep bugs at bay?" Consumer Reports, http://www.consumerreports.org/health/healthy-living/beauty-personal-care/personal-care/insect-repellents/insect-repellents-606/overview/index.htm.

Chapter 29 Rearrange Your Living Space

1. "Change," QuoteGarden.com, http://www.quotegarden.com/change.html.

2. *Pick the Brain*, "Does Your Brain Need an Oil Change?" February 13, 2008, http://www.pickthebrain.com/blog/brain-fitness/.

3. Barbara Riley, "Your Brain—Use it or Risk Losing It as You Age," Ohio Department of Aging, March 2009, http://aging.ohio.gov/news/agingissues/ai_2009_3a.asp.

4. Suzie Cortright, "Simple Feng Shui: Eight Quick Ways to Redecorate for Your Spirit." *All-Home Décor*, March 2004,: http://www.all-homedecor.com/fengshui.htm.

Chapter 30 Refuse to Retire

1. http://www.quotegarden.com/retirement.html.

2. Karla Freeman, "Don't Retire, Re-Invent!" My Article Archive, http://www.myarticlearchive.com/articles/7/176.htm.

3. Sue Poremba, "Another Shot: Reinventing Yourself After 60," *Grandparents Today*, http://www.grandparentstoday.com/articles/grandparent-leisure-time/another-shot-4421/.

4. Judy Shan, Tsai Wendt, Robin Donnelly, Geert de Jong, and Farah Ahmed, "Age at retirement and long term survival of an industrial population: prospective cohort study" (Pub Med, 2005), http://www.pubmed central.nih.gov/articlerender.fcgi?artid=1273451.

5. Brian Kurth, "Reinventing Yourself After Retirement," Vocation-vacations.com, http://vocationvacations.com/files/PDF/Reinventing_Your self_After_Retirement.pdf.

Chapter 31 Rejoice

1. "Single photon emission computed tomography," Wikipedia, http://en.wikipedia.org/wiki/Single_photon_emission_computed_ tomo graphy.

2. Earl Henslin, *This Is Your Brain on Joy* (Nashville: Thomas Nelson), 29.

3. Ibid., 39.

4. Ibid., 40.

Chapter 32 Replay Good Times

1. "Memory," Quotegarden.com, http://www.quotegarden.com/mem ory.html. *The Roadmender* was a huge success in its time, and is available today online at: http://www.gutenberg.org/etext/705.

2. Constantine Sedikides, et. al, "Nostalgia Isn't What it Used to Be," *Current Directions in Psychological Science* (17:5; 2008): 304. http://alt.coxnewsweb.com/shared-blogs/austin/health/upload/2008/12/nostalgia_ isnt_what_it_used_to/Sedikides-%20nostalgia%20current%20dir.pdf.

3. Ibid., 305.

4. Ibid., 306.

5. Mariya Simakova, "The Neurobiology of Nostalgia: A Story of Memory, Emotion, and the Self," Bryn Mawr College, 2002, http://ser endip.brynmawr.edu/bb/neuro/neuro06/web3/msimakova.html.

6. "More Than Just Being a Sentimental Fool: The Psychology of Nostalgia," *Science Daily* (December 14, 2008, http://www.sciencedaily.com/ releases/2008/12/081212141851.htm.

Chapter 33 Resolve Damaging Emotions

1. Mark Siegel, "The Irony of Fear," *The Washington Post*, August 30, 2005, http://www.washingtonpost.com/wp-dyn/content/article/2005/08/29/ AR2005082901391.html.

2. Ibid.

3. Timothy Stokes, "Got a Stubborn Psychological Problem? You Can Probably Blame it on Your Amygdala," *Psychology Today*, September 14, 2009, http://www.psychologytoday.com/blog/what-freud-didnt-know/ 200909/got-stubborn-psychological-problem-you-can-probably-blame-your-amy.

4. Doug Holt, "The Role of the Amygdala in Fear and Panic," *SerendipUpdate*, January 8, 2008, http://serendip.brynmawr.edu/exchange/ node/1749.

Chapter 34 Stay Focused

1. Adam J. Cox, "Understanding the Eight Pillars of Executive Control," http://concordspedpac.org/ExecutiveFunctions.html.

2. "Training Benefits Brains in Older People, Counters Aging Factors," *Medical News Today*, February 21, 2006, www.medicalnewstoday.com/ printerfriendlynews.php?newsid=37973.

3. "Exercise keeps your brain from deteriorating," *Medical News Today*, October 18, 2008, http://www.medicalnewstoday.com/printer friendlynews.php?newsid=125938.

4. "Executive Functions," http://en.wikipedia.org/wiki/Executive_ functions.

5. Michael Austin, "Texting While Driving: How Dangerous Is It?" *Car and Driver*, June 2009, http://www.caranddriver.com/features/09q2/ texting_while_driving_how_dangerous_is_it_-feature.

6. "Texting while driving," Wikipedia, http://en.wikipedia.org/wiki/ Texting_while_driving.

7. Adam J. Cox, *No Mind Left Behind: Why Executive Control Skills are Essential for Every Child—and How Parents and Educators Can Sharpen Them* (Penguin Book Group, 2007).

Chapter 35 Stay Socially Active

1. http://www.about-personal-growth.com/relationship-quotes.html.
2. "Taking Control of Brain Health: Stay Socially Connected," AARP, http://www.aarp.org/health/healthyliving/brain_health/articles/brain_so cially_connected.html.
3. Ibid.
4. Tom Valeo, "Good Friends are Good for You," WebMD, http://www.webmd.com/balance/good-life-health-well-being-9/friends-relation ships?print=true.
5. "Socialization," FitBrains, http://www.fitbrains.com/lifestyle/socialization.php.

Chapter 36 Stop Killing Your Brain with Your Fork

1. "Can Unhealthy Food Hijack Your Brain?" CBS News, http://cbs news.com/stories/2009/04/20/health/main4958349.shtml.
2. "Saturated Fats Can Cause Alzheimer's Disease," http://news-reviews.org/uncategorized/saturated-fats-can-cuase-alzheimers-disease/.
3. Information on this subject can be found at: http://en.wikipedia.org/wiki/Neurotoxicity.
4. Larry McCleary, "The Goldilocks Principle" (September 13, 2007), http://www.drmccleary.com/2007/09/13/TheGoldilocksPrinciple.aspx.
5. The name and story are fictitious, though doesn't the story sound oddly familiar?
6. "Obese People Have 'Severe Brain Degeneration'," *Live Science*, August 25, 2009, http://www.livescience.com/health/090825-obese-brain.html.
7. Various methods of figuring one's BMI (Body Mass Index) can be found online, including at: http://www.nhlbisupport.com/bmi/bminojs.htm.
8. McCleary, "Goldilocks Principle."

Chapter 37 Teach Your Brain to Tango

1. Greg Tanghe, *Pearls: Philosophies for Living a Robust and Fulfilling Life* (Andover, MN: Expert Publishing, 2004), 182.
2. "Keeping Fit Improves Spatial Memory, Increases Size Of Brain Structure," *Medical News Today*, February 25, 2009, http://www.medi calnewstoday.com/articles/140186.php.
3. Ibid.
4. Y. C. Peia, S. W. Choua, P. S. Linb, Y. C. Lina, T. H. Hsua, and A. M. Wonga, "Eye-hand Coordination of Elderly People Who Practice Tai Chi

Chuan," *Journal of the Formosan Medical Association* (107, Issue 2, February 2008): 103–10.

5. L. Baker, S. Craft, C. W. Wilkinson, P. Green, S. R. Plymate, G. S. Watson, B. Cholerton, L. Smith, and L. Fisher, "Six months of controlled aerobic exercise reduces cortisol for women but not men with MCI" *Alzheimer's and Dementia* (vol. 5, no. 4, supplement 1, July 2009): 334.

6. The Dana Foundation's homepage is: http://www.dana.org/default. aspx. Information about the study, including a download link is at: http://www.dana.org/news/publications/publication.aspx?id=10760.

7. "Learning, Arts, and the Brain," The Dana Consortium Report on Arts and Cognition, http://www.dana.org/uploadedFiles/News_and_Pub lications/Special_Publications/Learning,%20Arts%20and%20the%20 Brain_ArtsAndCognition_Compl.pdf.

Chapter 38 Tune In to Your Senses

1. http://www.brainyquote.com/quotes/keywords/senses.html.

2. "Aging Changes in the Senses," University of Maryland Medical Center (accessed February 19, 2009, http://www.umm.edu/ency/article/004013. htm).

3. Ibid.

4. Melissa Galea, "Brain Games," *Alive* (no. 297, July 2007), http://www.alive.com/6165a15a2.php?subject_bread_cramb=80.

5. "Aging Changes in the Senses," *Alive* (no. 297, July 2007), http://www.alive.com/6165a15a2.php?subject_bread_cramb=80.

6. Ibid.

7. Ibid.

8. "Proprioception," The Sound Learning Centre, http://www.the soundlearningcentre.co.uk/the-cause/proprioception-2/.

Chapter 39 Understand How Alcohol Affects Your Brain

1. See Quotesdaddy.com, http://www.quotesdaddy.com/quote/306969.

2. http://www.healthchecksystems.com/alcohol.htm. For more information on the work and resources of the National Council on Alcohol and Drug Dependence (an NIH affiliate) see: http://www.ncadd .org/.

3. A. Ruitenberg, et al, "Alcohol consumption and Risk of Dementia: The Rotterdam Study," *The Lancet* (359, no. 9303; 2002): 281–86.

4. "Using High-Tech Tools to Assess Alcoholic Brain Damage," *Alcohol Alert*, U.S. Department of Health and Human Services (63, October 2004): 3.

5. Ibid.

Chapter 40 Worship God in Spirit and Truth

1. Timothy R. Jennings, *Could It Be This Simple?* (Hagerstown, MD: Autumn House Publishing, 2007), 12.

2. See Acts 17:22 and following to discover how Paul leveraged the religiousness of the Athenians.

3. David B. Biebel, "Pulling Out the Hole," *Jonathan, You Left Too Soon* (Roseland, FL: Healthy Life Press, 2009).

David B. Biebel, DMin, is a minister, an award-winning author, a health educator, and editor of *Today's Christian Doctor*. He often speaks on health-related subjects and has been a guest on many radio and TV programs.

He may be reached by email at: DBBV1@AOL.COM. Visit his website at: http://www.crosshearthealth.com.

James E. Dill, MD, and Bobbie Dill, RN, were among the first husband-wife Christian medical teams to help establish a truly holistic medical practice. Jim is a board-certified gastroenterologist, and Bobbie is a nurse certified in women's health. Currently they reside temporarily in various places around the United States, from Massachusetts to Hawaii, as Jim provides locum tenens medical care, often for several months at a time.

Give Your "Blah" Mood the Boot!

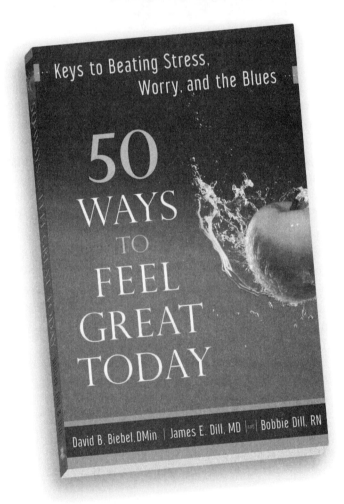

Start feeling better today with these medically sound and time-tested ideas to beat stress, ward off worry, and banish the blues.

You can have a brilliant mind— no matter what your age.

All your brain needs is a little exercise.

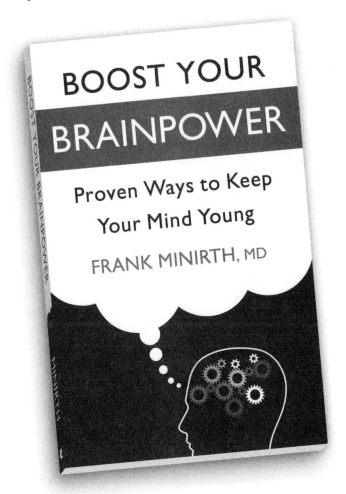

BOOST YOUR
BRAINPOWER
Proven Ways to Keep
Your Mind Young
FRANK MINIRTH, MD

Acclaimed psychiatrist and bestselling author Frank Minirth
will help you feel better, think better, and live better than ever before.

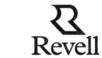